Community Psychology in Practice: An Oral History Through the Stories of Five Community Psychologists

Community Psychology in Practice: An Oral History Through the Stories of Five Community Psychologists has been co-published simultaneously as *Journal of Prevention & Intervention in the Community*, Volume 35, Number 1 2008.

Community Psychology in Practice: An Oral History Through the Stories of Five Community Psychologists

James G. Kelly
Anna V. Song
Editors

Community Psychology in Practice: An Oral History Through the Stories of Five Community Psychologists has been co-published simultaneously as *Journal of Prevention & Intervention in the Community*, Volume 35, Number 1 2008.

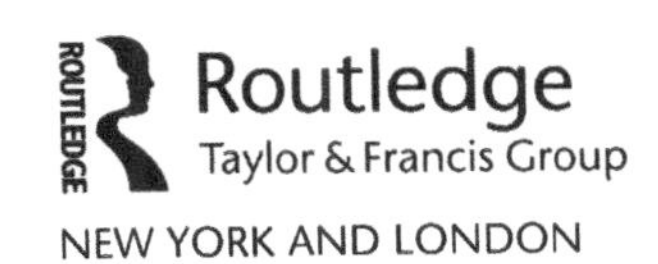

NEW YORK AND LONDON

First published 2008 by Haworth Press, Inc.

This edition published 2016 by Routledge
711 Third Avenue, New York, NY 10017, USA
2 Park Square, Milton Park, Abingdon, Oxon, OX14 4RN

Routledge is an imprint of the Taylor & Francis Group, an informa business

Community Psychology in Practice: An Oral History Through the Stories of Five Community Psychologists has been co-published simultaneously as *Journal of Prevention & Intervention in the Community®*, Volume 35, Number 1 2008.

Library of Congress Cataloging-in-Publication Data

Community psychology in practice : an oral history through the stories of five community psychologists / James G. Kelly, Anna V. Song, editors.
p. ; cm.
"Co-published simultaneously as Journal of prevention & intervention in the community, v. 35, no. 1, 2008."
Includes bibliographical references and index.
ISBN-13: 978-0-7890-3763-3 (hard cover : alk. paper)
ISBN-13: 978-0-7890-3764-0 (soft cover : alk. paper)
1. Community psychologists–United States–Biography. 2. Community psychology–United States–History. 3. Community mental health services–United States–History. I. Kelly, James G. II. Song, Anna V. III. Journal of prevention & intervention in the community.
[DNLM: 1. Community Psychiatry–United States–Personal Narratives. 2. Career Choice–United States–Personal Narratives. 3. Community Mental Health Services–United States–Personal Narratives. 4. Psychology, Social–United States–Personal Narratives. W1 PR497 v.35 no.1 2008 / WZ 112.5.P6 C734 2008]
RA790.55.C59 2008
362.2'0425–dc22

2007031306

ISBN 13:978-0-7890-3764-0 (pbk)

DEDICATION
TO
HENRY R. SCHEUNEMANN

A narrative is like a room on whose walls a number of false doors have been painted; while within the narrative, we have many apparent choices of exit, but when the author leads us to one particular door, we know it is the right one because it opens.

–John Updike

Community Psychology in Practice: An Oral History Through the Stories of Five Community Psychologists

CONTENTS

The Editors are grateful that the following gave feedback in conversations or on early drafts and offered substantive suggestions as well as support for this project: Paul Dolinko, Erin Hayes, Wendy Ho, Ming-Cheng Lo, John Morgan, Anne Mulvey, Gina Satin, Carol Schneider, Irma Serrano-García, Dan Romer, Steve Stelzner, Carolyn Swift, Rhona Weinstein, Bianca Wilson and Tom Wolff.

ABOUT THE EDITORS

James G. Kelly, PhD, is Emeritus Professor, University of Illinois at Chicago and now Research Associate, Department of Psychology, University of California at Davis. Dr. Kelly was the first elected President of Division 27 of the American Psychological Association in 1968, now the Society for Community Research and Action. In 1978 he received the award for Distinguished Contributions to Community Psychology and Community Mental Health from the Society. In 1997 he received the APA Senior Career Award for Distinguished Contributions to Psychology and the Public Interest. In 2001 he received the Seymour Sarason Award from the Society. He is Co-Author or Co-Editor of nine other books including the 2006 "Becoming Ecological: An Expedition into Community Psychology." He also has written on the history of community psychology including producing a DVD of early exemplars of the field.

Anna V. Song, PhD, is a postdoctoral fellow at the Center for Tobacco Control Research and Education at the University of California, San Francisco. Dr. Song received her doctorate in personality and social psychology at the University of California, Davis, writing her dissertation on cognitive style. Her two primary research interests are (1) methodological techniques in measuring personality characteristics including qualitative analyses and quantitative methods and (2) investigating how personality and culturally specific factors influence the decision-making process. Her research experience includes work in the field of political psychology with the Summer Institute for Political Psychology at Stanford University, the study of the History of Psychology as a Mountjoy graduate research fellow at the Archives for the History of American Psychology, research on addictive behaviors, and work with autobiographical narratives of leaders in the field of community psychology as published in the companion volume to the current book.

Introduction

Anna V. Song
James G. Kelly

SUMMARY. The current volume is comprised of five narratives representing the diverse spectrum of lives and careers in community psychology. The contributors to this book are exemplars of practitioners, activists, and researchers who have dedicated their careers to disseminating principles of community psychology. These community psychologists include Anne Mulvey, John Morgan, Irma Serrano-García, Tom Wolff, and Carolyn Swift. Their narratives touch upon themes related to autobiographical memory, family, careers, social class, ethnicity, and feminism. Jeremy Popkin, Roderick Watts, and Douglas Hall provide contextual background on all five narratives. It is the editors' hope that the work will provide an example of the diversity of paths the field of community psychology offers. doi:10.1300/J005v35n01_01 *[Article copies available for a fee from The Haworth Document Delivery Service: 1-800-HAWORTH. E-mail address: <docdelivery@haworthpress.com> Website: <http://www.HaworthPress.com>*

KEYWORDS. Autobiography, life stories, community psychology, careers, history of psychology

[Haworth co-indexing entry note]: "Introduction." Song, Anna V., and James G. Kelly. Co-published simultaneously in *Journal of Prevention & Intervention in the Community* (The Haworth Press) Vol. 35, No. 1, 2008, pp. 1-9; and: *Community Psychology in Practice: An Oral History Through the Stories of Five Community Psychologists* (ed: James G. Kelly, and Anna V. Song) The Haworth Press, 2008, pp. 1-9. Single or multiple copies of this article are available for a fee from The Haworth Document Delivery Service [1-800-HAWORTH, 9:00 a.m. - 5:00 p.m. (EST). E-mail address: docdelivery@haworthpress.com].

Available online at http://jpic.haworthpress.com

doi:10.1300/J005v35n01_01

INTRODUCTION

> One of the most important functions of narrative is to situate particular events against a larger horizon of what we consider to be human passions, virtues, philosophies, actions and relationships . . . Through narrative we come to know what it means to be a human being.
>
> –Ochs & Capps, 1996, pp. 30-31

The Conference on the Education of Psychologists for Community Mental Health held in Swampscott, MA in 1965 was a response to the growing national interest in having psychologists work in community mental health. The federal government, via the National Institute of Mental Health (NIMH), was very much interested in having psychologists work in community mental health. At the same time, independent of NIMH, there had been a growing number of psychologists who had been working at the community level since World War II (Wilson, Hayes, Greene, Kelly, & Iscoe, 2003; Kelly, 2005). These psychologists were for the most part dedicated to moving beyond strictly a focus on mental health services to issues of community development; moving away from a professional emphasis on diseases and the treatment of them. As phrased in the Swampscott conference report: "the point was emphasized that if psychology wants to make an impact on large social processes (and a majority of this sample of psychology accepted that goal), it will have to step out of its immersion in strictly clinical-medical settings" (Bennett et al., 1966, p. 5). Through a process of deliberation and advocacy a new field labeled "Community Psychology" was accepted within psychology in 1966.

As described in our companion volume (Kelly & Song, 2004) and other works such as Rickel (1987), Kelly (1987), and Shinn (1987), the ethos surrounding the Swampscott Conference in 1965 was to create a field dedicated to the training of psychologists with focus on action, intervention, and community development. This spirit is illustrated in the Swampscott conference's definition of a community psychologist: "Community psychologists were characterized as change agents, social systems analysts, consultants in community affairs, and students generally of the whole man [sic] in relation to all his environments" (Bennett et al., 1966, p. 26).

Even though the Swampscott definition of community psychology suggests an emphasis on applied values, a shared desire to establish university-based training for this new field and to be accepted as a scientific field led to a more visible focus on empirical research and evaluation, in contrast to direct community organizing. In actuality, the Swampscott participants were less dichotomous and they expressed hopes for a field where individuals could freely pass between both academic and applied activities. And although there has been a trend for careers to be developed inside or outside academe, there are few examples of moving between academic and applied settings. This volume presents five cases of such community psychologists. These examples are not only exemplar cases, they also highlight differences in career choices and experiences between academic and applied community psychologists.

There appear to be several differences in the career development of academic and applied community psychologists. To clarify this distinction, we call attention to the construct of *reference groups*. Research on reference groups was pioneered by Hyman (1942) and Sherif (1964). According to the theory, people tend to adopt the norms of a group for whom they respect. Subsequently, these individuals use these norms to evaluate themselves and others. It seems that community psychologists who enter the field as academics find readily available reference groups through mentors and influential colleagues within their departments and research units. Many of these researchers credit their intellectual and career developments to these key figures. Alternatively, as graduate students, applied community psychologists may find that reference groups are not as available within psychology for their applied and activist orientation; it may be more difficult to identify like-minded mentors and peers. This may be especially true for graduate students in primarily academic research-oriented programs. In this case, community psychologists with applied interests frequently embark to find groups who share their sense of activism, thus creating their own reference group.

Another distinction between academic and applied community psychology is the accessibility of information about the evolution of becoming a member of the field. As with many scientific fields, individuals working in academia have tangible outlets for their work such as publications in established journals or books. Academic career paths can be discerned through the researcher's publication history or through writings about their careers. In contrast, the professional evolution of applied community psychologists can be less visible. The paths to their current position may not be as easily discernable as the emphasis is less on publications and more on the design, implementation and maintenance of community-based services and programs. Therefore, psychologists entering the field of community psychology may be less likely to learn how one might become a "practicing" community psychologist. There are some illustrations of how practicing community psychologists go about defining their careers as in the commentaries of David Snow, the late Ruth Schelkun, Judith Meyers, Bill Berkowitz, David Chavis along with John Morgan, Carolyn Swift and Tom Wolff who also have included their autobiographical reports included in this volume (see Wolff, 2000). O'Donnell and Ferrari have also presented additional examples (O'Donnell & Ferrari, 2000).

THE CURRENT VOLUME

The impetus of this volume is to document a narrative history of the field from the perspective of community psychologists who navigated from academia to pursue applied careers. The contributors to this book are exemplars of practitioners, activists, and researchers who have dedicated their careers to disseminating principles of community psychology. These community psychologists include Anne Mulvey, John Morgan, Irma Serrano-García, Tom Wolff, and Carolyn Swift. In providing these narrative studies, it is our hope that younger and newer members of the field who have a goal other than a conventional academic career might find solace in the evolution of the careers of the five contributors.

Anne Mulvey, Professor of Psychology at the University of Massachusetts Lowell (UML), teaches women's studies and community psychology, integrating field work, feminist activism and creative expression into her courses. She has coordinated the UML Community Social Psychology Master's and Women's Studies programs, directed the campus Center for Diversity & Pluralism, and participated in many campus-community collaboratives. Anne has published theoretical, empirical, and creative writing related to her interests; served as National Coordinator and National Student Representative to the Society for Community Research and Action; and been recognized for her work by Fellowship in the American Psychological Association (APA) in APA Divisions 27, 35 and 44.

John Morgan has worked in the community mental health field for 30 years, first as founder and director of his center's prevention programs, and then as the Clinical Director. He has advanced the field of primary prevention through numerous articles, presentations, training and consulting activities, and policy and advocacy work at local, state and national levels. He is a fellow of the Society for Community Research and Action (APA Division 27), and the recipient of its Distinguished Practice Award (1990) and the McNeill Award for Innovation in Community Mental Health (1991).

Irma Serrano-García is a Puerto Rican social-community psychologist. She has devoted her life to facilitating the exchange between academic and applied settings while fostering the training of new professionals in the field. Her interests have varied as have the levels of interventions she engages in as a result of her own interests and the socio-historical context in which she is working. She is a past recipient of the SCRA Ethnic Minority Mentorship Award (1995). In 2005 she received the Award for Distinguished Contributions to Education and Training from the American Psychological Association.

Tom Wolff is a community psychologist and social justice activist committed to integrating a social change agenda into his work. Through Tom Wolff & Associates, a national consulting firm, he focuses on collaborative solutions, coalition building and community development. For his work, he was awarded the SCRA Distinguished Practice Award in 1985. The integration of a spiritual perspective into his work is the immediate challenge that now consumes his interest and energy.

Carolyn Swift is a community psychologist practitioner who has pioneered consultation in unconventional settings, including a Midwestern city hall and an interactive television station. Her career path has been shaped by events in her personal life–a 10-year hiatus to raise children, a commuting marriage, and family deaths–and by historical events, including two wars, the civil rights and women's movements, and the advances of technology. The application of prevention and empowerment theories are central themes in her work, with the prevention of rape and sexual abuse a priority focus. She is a recipient of the Distinguished Practice Award (1984) and is President-Elect of SCRA 2005-2006.

GUIDELINES FOR THE VOLUME

The pressures of academic cultures for community psychologists to conform to the traditional *modus operandi*, may be overwhelming for some who enter the field. Indeed, newcomers to the field may find it challenging to find support for subscribing to unorthodox methods, paradigms, or topics to work on. To highlight themes as they relate to their paths as applied community psychologists, the editors provided the five contributors with a set of brief guidelines. We asked them to think about several topics related to four experiential dimensions: **Personal, Contextual, Intellectual,** and **Ideological**. *Personal* dimensions refer to family and developmental antecedents that seem salient for their evolving career.

Contextual domains involve topics such as race, culture, class and circumstances that enabled the contributors to enter community psychology yet take an alternative path for creating a career. The *intellectual* dimension includes concepts, ideas and mentors who provided anchors and reference points during the evolution of their careers. Finally *ideological* topics are values, beliefs, and political views that inspired choices and decisions to seek out venues that were congruent with their individual sense of self. Each of the contributors referred to these broad categories when they made their statements. But we suggested that they not be constrained by them. Although each autobiographical narrative is different, the reader may see that each contributor weaves together the four domains.

AUTOBIOGRAPHICAL NARRATIVES: LEARNING LESSONS, CHALLENGING TRUTHS, AND FORMING IDENTITIES

Autobiographical narratives are a particularly effective medium to relay one's life story, though narratives are not without their methodological critics. Thus, as with most autobiographical work, there are certain assumptions that should be addressed. In particular, the issue of accuracy and objectivity of memories tends to arise when dealing with autobiographical material. Some scholars condemn autobiographical information as fallible, and unreliable. This perspective is encapsulated in Donnell's (1999) observation: "a genre autobiography can be likened to a restless and unmade bed; a site on which discursive, intellectual and political practices can be remade; a ruffled surface on which the traces of previous occupants can be uncovered and/or smoothed over" (p. 124).

It may be the case that autobiographical memory is susceptible to social construction, biases, and interpretations, but these "flaws" are just as informative and useful as "accurate" memories themselves. Pasupathi (2001) notes that autobiographical memory serves an important function in adult development. Rather than using a criteria based on accuracy, she promotes the principle of consistency: later recollections will influence the interpretations of earlier recollections. This, in turn, allows an individual to re-develop their identity and incorporate significant events in their lives. Alea and Bluck (2003) also stress the importance of autobiographical memories by proposing a conceptual model of autobiographical memory. Focusing on autobiographical memories that involve other people, memories can serve at least three important social functions. These functions include developing relationships, teaching others, eliciting empathy or providing support to others. It is apparent that the narratives included in this volume demonstrate each of these functions.

McAdams (1988, 1997, 2006) argues, people attach meaning to their lives by developing self-defining stories. In turn, these life stories become identities and their telling is an expression of who they are, where they came from, and how they arrived to the present point. Staudinger (2001) uses the term "life reflection" to describe the tendency to take overarching meaning through a process called *life review*. To engage in life reviews, people select incidents from their life story. These selected episodes are translated into self-defining memories (Singer, 2005, 2004). The re-telling of these self-defining stories then becomes the writers' attempt to share crystallizing events that changed their way of thinking (Singer & Bluck, 2001). As Eakin (2004) states: "Autobiography is not merely something we read in a book; rather, as a discourse of identity, delivered bit by bit in the stories we tell about ourselves day in and day out, autobiography structures our living" (p. 122). In other words, our contributors are not only providing an account of their lives, but as Cohler and Hammack (2006) argue, they are performing their identities through writing.

Wang and Brockmeier (2002) contribute an additional component to the conceptualization of autobiographical works. In addition to adopting the premise that the self is a running narrative and that autobiographies are presentations of identity, Wang and Brockmeier also argue that autobiographies are active social constructions that include the individual and both micro- and macro-environments. In the case of the current volume, autobiographical memories may represent "a cultural practice" akin to both academic and applied community psychology.

Nelson and Fivush (2004) add another dimension to the cultural practice perspective of autobiographical memory. They not only agree that autobiographical memory is necessarily tied to social cultural "milieu," but also argue that this type of memory is distinct from other forms of memory in terms of developmental emergence and its associated functions. Based on their extensive analysis, Nelson and Fivush propose autobiographical memory as a dynamic process involving self, identity, temporal constructs, mental concepts, language, and cognitive representations. Our contributors demonstrate these principles by revealing social constructions experienced in the past but recalled in the present day. Therefore, these "revelations" not only represent the actual experience, but also the experience as influenced by a lifetime of other experiences in the context of the individual's current self-identity, beliefs, and attitudes.

To provide a contextual background for you, the reader, we've asked several scholars, both inside and outside community psychology, to comment on these autobiographical reports. Jeremy D. Popkin, Professor of History at the University of Kentucky, has published *History, Historians and Autobiography* (University of Chicago Press, 2005) and several articles on academic autobiography. Rod Watts is a community and clinical psychologist, and a member of the psychology faculty at Georgia State University in Atlanta. His research and applied interests are in liberation psychology, men's development, and youth sociopolitical development. Douglas T. Hall, Professor of Organizational Behavior at Boston University, lends his expertise on career development and the integration between life and work domains.

The Editors hope that no matter what the level of the reader's interest in the field of community psychology, the words of the five contributors will inform the reader about the evolution and circumstances of creating a career. The Editors also intend that these reflections offer hope that a real and satisfying career can be obtained.

REFERENCES

Alea, N., & Bluck, S. (2003). Why are you telling me that? A conceptual model of the social function of autobiographical memory. *Memory, 11,* 165-178.

Bennett, C. C., Anderson, L. S., Cooper, S., Hassol, L., Klein, D. C., & Rosenblum, G. (1966). *Community psychology: A report of the Boston conference on the education of psychologists for community mental health.* Boston: Boston University.

Cohler, B. J., & Hammack, P. L. (2006). Making a gay identity: Developmental and cultural perspectives. In D. P. McAdams, R. Josselson, & A. Lieblich (Eds.), *Identity: Narrative studies of lives* (pp. 151-174). Washington, DC: American Psychological Association.

Donnell, A. (1999). When writing the other is being true to the self: Jamaica Kincaid's the autobiography of my mother. In P. Polkey (Ed.), *Women's lives into print: The theory, practice and writing of feminist auto/biography* (pp. 123-136). New York: St. Martin's Press.

Eakin, P. J. (2004). What are we reading when we read autobiography? *Narrative, 12*(2), 121-132.

Hyman, H. H. (1942). The psychology of status. *Archives of Psychology, 269,* 5-91.

Kelly, J. G. (1987). Some reflections on the Swampscott conference. *American Journal of Community Psychology, 15,* 515-517.

Kelly, J. G. (2005). The National Institute of Mental Health and the founding of the field of community psychology. In W. E. Pickren & S. F. Schneider (Eds.), *Psychology and the National Institute of Mental Health* (pp. 233-259). Washington, DC: American Psychological Association.

Kelly, J. G., & Song, A. V. (Eds.) (2004). *Six community psychologists tell their stories: History, context, and narratives.* New York: The Haworth Press.

McAdams, D. P. (2006). *The redemptive self: Stories Americans live by*. Oxford University Press.

McAdams, D. P. (1997). *Stories we live by: Personal myths and the making of the self*, 2nd ed. London: Guilford Press.

McAdams, D. P. (1988). *Power, intimacy, and the life story: Personological inquiries into identity*. New York: Guilford Press.

Nelson, K., & Fivush, R. (2004). The emergence of autobiographical memory: A social cultural developmental theory. *Psychological Review, 111*, 486-511.

O'Donnell, C. R., & Ferrari, J. R. (Eds.) (2000). *Employment in community psychology: The diversity of opportunity*. New York: The Haworth Press.

Pasupathi, M. (2001). The social construction of the personal past and its implications for adult development. *Psychological Bulletin, 127*, 651-672.

Rickel, A. U. (1987). The 1965 Swampscott conference and future topics for Community Psychology. *American Journal of Community Psychology, 15*, 511-513.

Sherif, M., & Sherif, C. W. (1964). *Reference groups: Exploration into conformity and deviation of adolescents*. New York: Harper and Row.

Shinn, M. (1987). Expanding community psychology's domain. *American Journal of Community Psychology, 15*, 555-574.

Singer, J. A. (2005). *Memories that matter: Using self-defining memories to understand and change your life*. Oakland, CA: New Harbinger.

Singer, J. A. (2004). Narrative identity and meaning-making across the adult span: An introduction. *Journal of Personality, 72*, 437-459.

Singer, J. A., & Bluck, S. (2001). New perspectives on autobiographical memory: The integration of narrative processing and autobiographical reasoning. *Review of General Psychology, 5*, 91-99.

Staudinger, U. M. (2001). Life reflection: A social-cognitive analysis of life review. *Review of General Psychology, 5*, 148-160.

Wang, Q., & Brockmeier, J. (2002). Autobiographical remembering as cultural practice: Understanding the interplay between memory, self and culture. *Culture & Psychology, 8*, 45-64.

Wilson, B. D., Hayes, E., Greene, G. J., Kelly, J. G., & Iscoe, I. (2003). Community psychology. In D. K. Freedheim & I. B. Weiner (Eds.), *Handbook of psychology: Vol. I. History of psychology*. Hoboken, NJ: Wiley.

Wolff, T. (Ed.) (2000). Practitioners' perspectives. In J. Rappaport & E. Seidman (Eds.). *Handbook of community psychology* (pp. 741-777). New York: Kluwer-Academic.

doi:10.1300/J005v35n01_01

Reconceiving Myself: Challenging Conundrums and Creating Feminist Community Psychology

Anne Mulvey

University of Massachusetts Lowell

SUMMARY. This narrative describes how contexts in which I grew up influenced my pursuit of feminist community psychology and my work in a master's level community psychology program. Grappling inside and outside with longings that appear contradictory and contradictions that others do not experience has fueled passionate engagement with life and work. Growing up an Irish Catholic girl in the Midwest U.S. post World War II era informed and constrained my relational and vocational choices. Participation in consciousness raising and informal community building initiatives opened opportunities for personal, professional and political growth. These intensely personal interconnected stories describe conundrums that I experienced and the ways in which they were

---

Anne Mulvey is affiliated with the Department of Psychology, University of Massachusetts Lowell.

The author wishes to thank Donna O'Neill, her spouse, and Irene Egan, Miriam Klein, Kathy Desilets, Pat Schneider, Elizabeth Thomas and Charlotte Mandell for their great editing, suggestions, and ongoing support.

Address correspondence to: Anne Mulvey, Department of Psychology, University of Massachusetts, 870 Broadway Street, Lowell, MA 01854 (E-mail: anne_mulvey@uml.edu).

[Haworth co-indexing entry note]: "Reconceiving Myself: Challenging Conundrums and Creating Feminist Community Psychology." Mulvey, Anne. Co-published simultaneously in *Journal of Prevention & Intervention in the Community* (The Haworth Press) Vol. 35, No. 1, 2008, pp. 11-27; and: *Community Psychology in Practice: An Oral History Through the Stories of Five Community Psychologists* (ed: James G. Kelly, and Anna V. Song) The Haworth Press, 2008, pp. 11-27. Single or multiple copies of this article are available for a fee from The Haworth Document Delivery Service [1-800-HAWORTH, 9:00 a.m. - 5:00 p.m. (EST). E-mail address: docdelivery@haworthpress.com].

Available online at http://jpic.haworthpress.com

doi:10.1300/J005v35n01_02

reconceived and repaired in the process of creating self, work and community. doi:10.1300/J005v35n01_02 *[Article copies available for a fee from The Haworth Document Delivery Service: 1-800-HAWORTH. E-mail address: <docdelivery@haworthpress.com> Website: <http://www.HaworthPress.com>*

KEYWORDS. Feminist community psychology, social justice, spirituality

INTRODUCTION

I'm nobody! Who are you?/Are you nobody, too?

–Emily Dickinson

Writing a life narrative is a daunting task. I harbor a lifelong desire to be part of a decidedly romanticized notion of "one big happy family" in which each of us is deeply loved, has enough and chooses to share everything with everybody. This coexists with a desire to be recognized, singled out as uniquely special, and loved for myself alone. Grappling with longings that appear to be contradictory and with contradictions apparent to me that others do not experience has fueled passionate engagement with life and work. My journey has been accompanied by fear and uncertainty and by immense satisfaction, love and joy. Anticipating self-disclosure, I move toward the delete button when Audre Lorde tells me to go on despite fear since "most of all . . . we fear the visibility without which we cannot truly live" (1984, p. 42). What follows is the current version of how becoming me in my family and as a Catholic girl in the Midwest U.S. post World War II era affected choices, opening up and constraining opportunities that led to more than 25 years of doing feminist community psychology in a master's program in a mid-sized mill town similar to and different from the one I called home.

ONE BIG HAPPY FAMILY

Shamrocks and leprechauns, wee fairies in the wood/Irish need not apply, know your place and be good/Shanty or lace curtain, we were never certain . . .[1]

My family was and wasn't the big happy family that I thought we were and wanted us to be. Symmetrical and discordant threads of idyllic experiences and opportunities, contradictory values and practices, and themes of unworthiness and entitlement, were tightly interwoven into the fabric of my large middle-class Irish Catholic clan. The small settings and large socio-historical contexts that framed my youth were radically different from those of later life adding unexpected conundrums, revisions and repairs.

Beginnings

I was born in 1946 in Cleveland, Ohio, after my mother had had a spontaneous later term abortion. The nuns nursing her said that the abortion was a blessing and the doctor told her that she would be unable to conceive again. I was born just two years and nine months after my older sister Ellen; two weeks later my mother's brother died of a heart attack. My brother Billy was born when I was two; six months later my mother's mother died. Over the next nine years, my mother had another miscarriage followed by her father's death and the births of my brother Michael and my sisters Cate and Terry, respectively.

How hard it must have been for Mother living far away from family and friends to have three children under five and to lose her mother and brother. [2] *Until my brother Michael died when we were adults, I had no idea what grief felt like, but I had realized that my beginnings were marked by my mother's uprooting and losses. Being second, wanting to be first and being taught that wanting anything–especially to be first–was selfish, presented dilemmas and a desire to befriend those who were left out. Going to a convent high school from ages 14 to 17 was related to these dilemmas, as was deciding at age 10 or 11 to become a missionary nun.*

I grew up in Mishawaka, Indiana, a small city contiguous with South Bend of Notre Dame football fame. I was a Midwesterner, but my parents were not. My father left Brooklyn during World War II to be a supervisor in a munitions factory; my mother joined him when they married. My mother maintained close ties with family and friends. My father was less attached to his roots, but had colleagues from the east. I envied friends who had family reunions with 50 to 100 relatives. We spent holidays with other "transplants," some of whom were like family.

I liked going to Brooklyn and to the ocean to ride waves, play skeet ball and watch the pizza man toss dough high in the air, catching it every time. I loved visiting St. Patrick's Cathedral, the Statue of Liberty and the United Nations, symbols of compassion, belonging and community. What I liked most, though, was being part of an extended family.

Reflecting on what I thought was the difference between family and "like" family, a line from Robert Frost's "Death of the hired man," comes to mind: "Home is the place where, when you have to go there, / They have to take you in" (1979, p. 38). With that belonging comes the possibility of permanence and acceptance even of those who do not share interests or values.

Many Americans loved Frank McCourt's gripping autobiography of growing up in Limerick, but Mother hated *Angela's Ashes* (1996). The Irish could not have been that poor or mad or mean! My mother's family emigrated before the famine to escape religious persecution; we grew up with stories of ancestors sneaking out to the woods to "hear" silent Masses. From both sides we learned that "No Irish need apply" signs greeted "us." We were "dyed in the wool Democrats" . . . "on the side of the underdog." I embraced a distant past of persecution, poverty.

I went to my first St. Patrick's Day Parade in Chicago during college, was shocked at the drinking and vulgarity, and hated being teased and touched by men. Years later, I was angry but not shocked when the Boston St. Patrick's Day Parade Committee excluded gay organizations.

Who do you think you are? Growing up, the rhetorical question, "Who do you think you are?" was often posed to challenge pretension. The question was complicated for me. We lived in a working class neighborhood with little talk of class or status. We were the last family to get a television and had the most children, so I thought we were poor. Later, I found out that Mother wanted a piano and didn't want a TV in the living room. We got a piano, a den and then a TV. My father's stories strengthened my conviction that the poor deserve respect. An only child whose father died when he was about six, my father called himself an orphan by which he meant he did not remember his father. "Daddy's" eyes filled with tears when he repeated his mother's words: "Don't ever forget you're just a poor Irish boy from Brooklyn." I idolized my father and was sad that he had felt like an orphan, like a "nobody."

The work that I do stems from feelings of being second and the belief that no person should feel less than another. I learned that it was bad to be proud of self but good to be proud of family, culture, religion. Early messages that I should be and do good, but should not feel good about myself, are interwoven with later learning that doing good may be self-serving and destructive. Community psychology and feminism offered opposing and convergent perspectives that helped me to unpack, re-conceive and repair this conundrum.

I was shocked to learn that my mother had had another last name; I didn't understand how anyone could change something so central to identity. Knowing that women did, but men did not, led to questions about fairness.

The responses–"Tradition" and "Don't you want us all to have the same name?"–were not convincing. I knew children were not supposed to question adults, but it was hard not to voice opinions about things that mattered, and lots of things did.

Parental roles: Family, work, church and community. On the surface, the roles that my parents played were typical of the fifties. While my mother was the top math student in high school and college and loved numbers, she majored in history because she didn't think that math was feminine enough. After marrying at age 27, she did not seek paid work again. Informal roles that my parents had, however, were at odds with typical gendered division of labor. My mother learned to drive before my father did and was the better driver. Though my father was a traveling salesman and later flew all over the world, he was bad with directions. My mother handled finances and loved balancing the checkbook that served as our family archive.

In contrast to my father's emotional expressiveness, my mother was formal and reserved except with family and close friends. Grateful for his large family of six children, my father often called himself "a millionaire six times over"; Mother would respond, "I'll take the money." Not nurturing in the usual sense, my mother was extremely intelligent, knowledgeable, and disciplined; and she had a great sense of humor.

My family continues to hold a central place in my heart and life. As a child I loved my big happy family not realizing until much later that I may not have gotten the attention that I wanted, needed, or deserved. Distinguishing among the three has been hard. Most of the students with whom I work are women, many of whom learned as I did to consider the needs of others before their own. Seeing graduates contribute to our community in diverse ways and witnessing their personal transformations and professional growth has been wonderful.

Invisibility and visibility of race, rights and wrongs. My earliest memory of race concerns a nursery rhyme that begins, "Eanie meanie miney mo . . ." Instead of tiger, I heard children use another word. My mother told me the other word was "bad" and not ever to say it. I thought all adults would correct children and instead was shocked when I heard adults use it.

When I was five or so, the "egg man" came to our front door every Saturday to sell us eggs. We called him by his last name and, though he stayed only a few minutes, we asked him how his family was. He was white and went to our church. The "cleaning woman" came to our back door once a week. We called her by her first name, Leona. She stayed much longer and had lunch with us, but we rarely asked her about her family. She was black and didn't go to our church. I thought the differences might have to do with selling versus cleaning or with going to the same church, but I knew it also had to do with the color of skin, a thing called "race."

TV played a role in my experience of the violence of race. Watching coverage of non-violent civil rights protests was riveting. I watched dogs snarling and attacking people and the police aiming huge hoses of water full force at people who wanted the same rights I thought all Americans had. I learned that "colored people" weren't allowed to drink from the same water fountains as white people and some laws like who could vote were different in the south. Around that time, I asked my mother how she would feel if I married someone of another race. Her response was atypically vague.

Earlier I had asked questions about the Catholic Church. Even though my parents placed a high value on objective truth, they did not question inconsistencies in doctrines that I found troubling. With their encouragement, I accepted things on faith and embraced the spirit of religion which, for me, was unconditional love. When the family knelt down to pray for world peace with our matching rosaries, experiences of familial and global community were palpable. Each set of 10 beads was a different color to represent a continent and its people. I was praying to end war, feed the hungry, and "wipe out the red threat" of communism. I was also praying for eternal salvation, the greatest gift, which was only possible if you practiced one religion: ours.

Through early adulthood I had a personal relationship with Jesus that provided feelings of safety and belonging; I sometimes felt a cosmic connection singing sweet songs to Mary, but Jesus embodied spirituality for me. Jesus cared for the poor, the sick. Jesus spoke out against hypocrisy. Jesus died for all of us, even me. Mary was just a vessel, an old-fashioned word for box. The far-removed possibility of spiritual salvation through a trinity of male gods left little room for me and precluded participation in valued "earthly" roles for people like me. Denial and denigration of the body was pervasive in cultural and religious traditions. While I cherish memories of being part of one big happy family that stretched from our home to the world, I shudder at my colonial, misogynist and spiritual beliefs. The resultant devaluing of parts of my self and my own longing for loving communities have influenced my visions for community psychology. Repairing deep internal schisms has been hard and is my most challenging work.

HIGH SCHOOL: "COMING OUT," GOING IN, COMING OUT

"All for God the little way"

(Motto, Ancilla Domini High School, Class of 1964)

I had a hard time "coming out" about my choice of high choice, a small tuition free boarding school for girls who planned to join the Poor Handmaids of Jesus Christ, a German religious order with its main Motherhouse (headquarters) in Dusseldorf, and the only other in rural Indiana. I didn't tell my parents because they would not want me to leave home. I didn't tell peers for fear of appearing less interesting than I already did. I dreaded my choice becoming public for different reasons with different groups I was trying to please. I "came out," however, and "went in" to Ancilla Domini High School where I lived for three years excluding summers.

"Coming out" is typically seen as unidirectional, and refers only to those of us who disclose publicly for the first time that we do not identify as heterosexual. But coming out is a complicated concept useful for understanding the process involved in what a person chooses to disclose, to whom, and why. While a junior untenured faculty member, I began to discover an aspect of identity that was non-normative and not socially valued. The memory of how hard it had been to disclose a valued non-normative choice to attend a convent school buffered my coming out as a lesbian. With close friends, I came out quickly. With others, I sometimes came out when they made homophobic remarks as if they were not talking about me. Creating safe, welcoming places played a central role in pursuing community psychology, in becoming a feminist, and in my desires to be a missionary and a nun.

The summer between junior and senior years, I was asked to reconfirm my decision to enter the "Poor Handmaids," a teaching order. I was asked to leave when I "came out" with my desire to be a missionary. Coming out was harder than going in. Feelings of stigma and failure were strong. Back home, my 7th grade teacher was the only nun who spoke to me. At the time, my brother Bill was in a seminary preparing to be a priest. Sister Genevieve said: "God works in strange and wondrous ways. Maybe someday you'll be Billy's housekeeper." I knew that she meant well, but being my little brother's housekeeper would never have crossed my mind!

I experienced extreme culture shock during my senior year as a day student at a private boarding school that friends from grade school and I called "Snob Hill." I heard words like "damn" and had no idea what

"French kiss" meant. Academic expectations and demands were even more challenging. Meeting Dorothy Day was a highlight that year. I sat in my new school and listened to a woman I knew of from my father who greatly admired her. The founder of the Catholic Workers Movement, a progressive activist organization, she talked about poverty in our country and ways to end it. Dorothy Day confirmed that socialist and Catholic philosophies were, or at least could be, compatible. When she smiled at me and shook my hand, I smiled, too.

Leaving the convent school and, later, the Church was associated with dissociation from experiences of power, beauty and community. Feminism had appeal because it challenged disembodied intellectualism and patriarchal systems and valued emotions and lived experience. Feminist theories helped me to see that some groups were categorized as emotional, not rational, and as physical, not spiritual, and devalued using interrelated social systems and constructions, including institutionalized religion and concepts associated with rationalism and with spirituality.

COLLEGE: THE SIXTIES, BUT MORE LIKE THE FIFTIES

> *As a woman, I have no country. As a woman, the entire world is my country.*
>
> –Virginia Woolf

When I went to Barat College of the Sacred Heart in 1964, it was the sixties but more like the fifties. We were not allowed to wear slacks to meals or to classes; we all knelt outside of our rooms at 9:30 for night prayers. My college years raised questions about religion, politics, community and epistemology. Mother Maxey, who taught the required first semester theology class, asserted that the bible was an allegory, not literally true. This assertion from a nun exuding intelligence and confidence encouraged new ways of interpreting religion. Thomas Kuhn's book, *The Structure of Scientific Revolutions*, had a similar impact upon me in relation to the subjective, political nature of scientific paradigms, objectivity and truth (1970).

Martin Luther King, Stokely Carmichael . . . and me?

As a result of volunteering to tutor, college for me was bracketed by the life and death of Martin Luther King. We arrived to tutor in a Chicago neighborhood as usual and were told to hurry down the street to hear Dr. King! Seeing him in a church overflowing with people and positive energy deepened my commitment to social justice. This was my first experience as one of few whites in a large gathering of people of color, but I felt at home in a shared community.

For three years, I worked as a dorm mother, recreation counselor, and tutor in our campus Upward Bound Program with teen women from Chicago's South Side. During that time, Stokely Carmichael spoke on our campus; he told us to "go home," take care of our own communities and let black people take care of theirs. Though I didn't know where my community was, I knew that trying to "do good" was a way of trying to care for self. I felt confused and homeless.

During my last semester of college, Martin Luther King was assassinated. Some friends and I drove all night to attend his funeral. Marching in the funeral procession brought back memories of the power and possibility that I had felt when I heard Dr. King preach during my first semester. But this was sad and somber and I was personally and politically lost.

THE REAL WORLD: SCHOOL OF HARD KNOCKS

We have all known the long loneliness and we have learned that the only solution is love and that love comes with community.

–Dorothy Day (1952)

Experiencing "Hard Knocks" of Daily Living

Through college, I lived in small, relatively safe, middle-class settings. When I moved to San Francisco for a year and then to New York, I was not prepared for the post-baccalaureate "School of hard knocks." My training began with the discovery that all women (but not men) were required to take typing tests. Despite flunking, I was hired as a clerical worker. During a probation period without health insurance, I needed major surgery. My father had me reinstated on his insurance and paid for a plane ticket, so that I could fly "home" for surgery. *He was able to do that since he had a job that allowed him to "pull strings" and "bend the rules."*

Back in San Francisco, I found a better clerical job and started taking graduate courses. A month or so later, my apartment was shaking. We were having an earthquake and I imagined being swept into the ocean. I quit my job, dropped the courses and moved east to be closer to my family.

I worked for the New York City Public Housing Authority as a combination social worker/landlord in the Jacob Riis and Frederick Douglass projects, both large complexes.

In the year that I lived in San Francisco, my college friend Sue and I "crashed" on a friend's floor until we found a studio apartment, then moved when we couldn't afford the rent. In New York working in a professional job in public housing, I couldn't find affordable housing, so I "doubled up" with family alternating between my sister in Manhattan, an aunt in Brooklyn and my parents in Connecticut. After renting a 5th floor "walk-up" apartment, I was displaced by a fire; my family took me in again until I moved in with friends and discovered in November that we were living illegally in an unheated commercially zoned space. Desperate, I took a job as a nanny and rushed from my "real" job to pick up two little girls from daycare, walk home, make supper, and spend "quality time" with them before cajoling them to bed. An unintended consequence of this period is an inordinately increased appreciation of people who manage to survive without economic, social or familial supports that I took for granted (and still do).

When a public housing co-worker invited me to a women's consciousness-raising group, I hesitated, feeling more like a convent school girl than a "flower child" or radical, but later was glad that I went. The women's movement offered critical analytical tools, experiences of small and large community, and alternatives to the good girl "do-gooder." Though I could not prevent all of sexism's "hard knocks," I could name, revise and repair some. "Sisterhood was powerful!"

Experiencing "Hard Knocks" of Sexism

In different forms across time and place, I have had unwanted experiences with men of varied ages and cultural traditions. Ranging from normative and legal to non-normative and illegal, I believe that these experiences fall along a continuum that normalizes dominance by men and obscures misogyny. I have been told I would be prettier if I smiled, touched by strangers, kissed by bosses, mugged, robbed at gunpoint and sexually assaulted. The first incident that I remember (I was about seven) happened while I was riding my bike when something caught my eye; I looked and saw a man staring at me, holding his penis. I knew that I was not supposed to see this or to talk about what I saw. I told no one.

We need more "coming out" about the origins, extent and damage of sexism. The precursors of gendered violence, many of which are normative, greatly interest me. When women and girls share stories in supportive settings, it opens up possibilities for powerful insights, healing and activism. Many students are interested in violence against women because of their own experiences which suggests how important it is to provide opportunities for personal stories to be told, critically analyzed, and collectively transformed. My work in this area stems from a desire to provide information and support to others that I wish I could have had.

As a result of friendships formed in the consciousness-raising group, I moved to Brooklyn (Park Slope) where a group of us (women and men) formed the Community Group. We debated the utility of dense theories and attended to minute aspects of practice. After failed attempts to reach the "community" (poor people and people of color), we decided to create something that we ourselves would like, a coffee house called The Mongoose. We offered progressive cultural and political programs. The Park Slope Food Co-op which started there is now over 30 years old, owns the building, and "is the largest wholly member-owned and operated food co-op in the country" (www.foodcoop.com/PSFC/retrieved 08/26/05).

GRADUATE SCHOOL: FROM GENERAL TO SOCIAL TO COMMUNITY PSYCHOLOGY

The white fathers told us: I think, therefore I am. The Black mother whispers in our dreams: I feel, therefore I can be free.

–Audre Lorde (1984, p. 38)

"Terminal" Master's: Intellectual or Elitist Problem?

After working in public housing for a few years, I enrolled in the General Psychology Program at Hunter College, City University of New York (CUNY). When I sought permission to take the Psychology of Women, a new doctoral course being taught by my social psychology instructor Florence Denmark, the department chair said that I was in a "terminal" master's program and questioned my ability. I feigned confidence; the course was great. In 1973, thanks to Florence's encouragement and success in the course, I began doctoral work in the Social Personality Program at the CUNY Graduate Center. The urban psychology sub-program was a better fit for my interests than the program in which it was embedded. Morton Bard and Barbara Dohrenwend co-led the program. Great role models, advisors and professional leaders, they were enthusiastic about the new field and created a setting within a setting.

Experiences in the master's program prepared me somewhat for the elitism in academia. I returned to graduate school to learn about the kinds of micro and macro systems that I valued. I wanted to work with people who had limited access to elite institutions not realizing that I was entering a hierarchical system that valued research above all and often accorded star status to individuals based on criteria that I did not value. Many students come to our master's program on a non-matriculated basis, and some use it as a stepping stone to doctoral programs. I tested the waters by taking courses in two programs, matriculating in a third, and taking a doctoral course in a fourth! My interest in the job at UMass Lowell (formerly the University of Lowell), however, had to do with the job description, not the program level or type of institution. My circuitous career path, experiences of elitism in academia, questioning of my potential, and appreciation of teachers who encouraged me from nursery school on, all contributed to my commitment to teaching undergraduate and master's students at a public institution.

Discovering Community Psychology

Barbara Snell Dohrenwend: Little things mean a lot. Before I met Barbara Dohrenwend, she called to offer me a National Institute of Mental Health pre-doctoral fellowship on the basis of the experiences and goals that I described in my doctoral application; she was the first teacher ever to call me. When I met her at an event for new students, she asked about my family, not professional interests. We found common ground in our experiences living away from home in "all girl" high schools. She shared her past in ways that welcomed me. Later, when I asked her to supervise my thesis on a feminist topic, she responded with a refreshing variation on "I'm not a feminist, but . . . ," saying that she didn't think she had done enough politically to have *earned* the label. Barbara was, however, the first woman president of the Division of Community Psychology of the American Psychological Association/APA (Div. 27, now the Society for Community Research and Action/SCRA); she was also the first woman to receive the Division's Distinguished Contributions Award (with her husband Bruce). She was extremely intelligent and productive. I was drawn to Barbara for these reasons and because she was kind.

The Austin Conference: Far better and far worse. As a second year doctoral student, I participated in the Austin training conference. Marking the 10th anniversary of the founding of the field, the purpose was to define and evaluate community psychology training models. I participated in a social change model group facilitated by Margie Gatz and

Ramsey Liem. Meeting community psychologists passionately committed to creating socially just communities and excited by critical, multi-level analyses, I was "hooked" on the new field. Unfortunately, in large sessions, speakers used sexist language and told sexist jokes. Discussing experiences of women at the conference, Leidig (1977, p. 274) noted: "We . . . heard numerous jokes at our expense (e.g., 'community psychology needs new girlfriends'), and when we expressed disdain at these kinds of comments, some of us were told to 'not take things so seriously'. Paternalistic hugs and pats were also evident." These practices were not common in my networks and I did not expect to find them in a field like community psychology.

On the last day of the conference, the training model groups presented summaries with no mention of women's issues. In small groups we made lists of issues that we wanted for future consideration. I said that "women" should be on the list; the recorder said this was too negative. Noting that it was a group list, I repeated my request which was again denied; the list was collected. I hesitated for a long moment. It took every ounce of courage I had to stand up and to walk to the stage where the lists were. Shaking, I wrote "women as a constituent group." I felt an arm around me; a hand erased what I had written; a man was telling me that there was no problem, and I had nothing to worry about. I said I disagreed, but I did not re-write my words or challenge his inappropriate touching.

Though a feminist activist, I was still an easily intimidated good girl who wanted to be liked and was afraid to challenge authority. My commitment to feminist community psychology began in that moment experiencing personal and political erasure so soon after the euphoria of finding what I hoped would be a community where a good girl and feminist would find a home.

When I told Barbara what had happened, she encouraged me to run for election as national student representative to Division 27 and to propose to do a special issue of the *Journal of Community Psychology.* I agreed to run for office, but editing a journal issue seemed beyond my capacity. I was elected in 1976; as it turned out, being elected led to a special issue. Chairing a meeting in California as national student representative, I learned that Ann Mamo (D'Ercole), a doctoral student at New York University (NYU), and Rima Blair, a recent NYU graduate on the Staten Island Community College faculty, were interested in women's issues. Shared interests led to creating an informal group, mostly of students, where we discussed our work. Hearing that many advisors discouraged feminist work, I felt even luckier to work with Barbara and Mort. *I continue to hear that some advisors discourage and/or disparage research on feminist topics, and on lesbian, gay, bisexual and trans-gendered topics.*

Students are still shocked and disappointed as I was. We did a study that found few articles on women's issues had been published in community psychology journals (Blair, D'Ercole, O'Connor, Green, & Mulvey, 1978). In 1978, I presented our findings and recommendations to the Divisions 27 Executive Committee, and the Task Force on Women was established. I was the Psychology of Women (APA Div. 35) liaison to Division 27, so I offered to be the Division 27 liaison to Division 35. The dual role provided support for feminist work. Ann, Rima and I later co-edited a special issue of the *Journal of Community Psychology* (Mulvey, D'Ercole & Blair, 1988) in which was published my feminist critique of the field that I outlined the week after defending my dissertation (Mulvey, 1988). These experiences strengthened my commitment to the field.

LOWELL: CREATING COMMUNITIES INSIDE AND OUTSIDE

> *Urban gardens can be hard places to grow . . . /but sweetest of shoots replace other kinds . . .*

While finishing my dissertation, I took a research job at New York University's Medical Center and did not plan to leave my friends or neighborhood. When Kathy Grady, a friend from graduate school, and Nancy Henley, a friend from the Association for Women in Psychology, both told me that a job at the University of Lowell would be "perfect" for me, I applied despite my reservations about academia. Less than a year after receiving my degree I arrived in Lowell, was appointed assistant graduate coordinator, and was told to recruit students since the program must begin in two weeks or risk losing funding (I was elected coordinator the second year). We began with two courses and seven students as a group of faculty collaborated to develop a training program that used the city as a "learning lab." Designed for non-traditional students, we made no distinction between matriculated and non-matriculated students and offered classes only in the late afternoon and evening. Nancy had suggested that I call two people to find out about the city: Bill Berkowitz and Kathy Desilets have become my life-long friends. As her practicum project, Brinton Lykes helped us to develop our training model; her support came at a critical time in my and the program's development. Ramsey Liem was her academic supervisor which helped to connect me and the program to professional networks. Both the program and I celebrated our 25th anniversaries in 2005.

CONCLUSION: LOOKING BACK, MOVING FORWARD

Home is where the heart is/And there's no place like home.

"Life begins at 40" or "saving the best for last" would be appropriate headings for this section. Donna O'Neill has been at the center of my heart and family for almost 20 years since we met through a mutual friend when I was 40. Conundrums related to desires to live for myself and to live for community have deepened my gratitude and happiness that Donna Lee Jean O'Neill and I have created a family together.

In 2004, Donna and I publicly affirmed our love when we claimed our right to marry after Massachusetts legalized same-sex civil marriage. Happily, our given and chosen families celebrated our marriage with us. Experiencing new civil rights and public affirmation has strengthened my spirit even as backlash has exposed deep hatred and homophobia within many religions, political groups, and governments. Choosing to be married after not having the right to marry is a multi-layered affirmation of my self, of our relationship as uniquely special, and of families and communities as most deeply rooted in love and social justice.

The last time that I saw Barbara Dohrenwend was at a party at her house during my first or second year in Lowell. As I was leaving, she called me aside to tell me how glad she was that I was working in the Lowell program, and that I was her only student teaching community psychology. For an internationally renowned epidemiologist of her stature to affirm my work as a teacher meant a lot. In 1982 at the age of 55, Barbara died of cancer. I am older than she was then, but Barbara still serves as mentor, wise woman, and friend.

My family of origin experienced great losses from 1994 to 2004 with the death of my brother Michael (at age 42) and my father and mother, respectively. Losing them was awful, but the periods of illness and grieving were filled with much generosity and a psychological sense of community. We collaborated to provide, obtain and monitor medical, social and psychological services and willingly practiced the communist principle "from each according to their abilities, to each according to their needs." In the eulogy that I gave for my father, I quoted him: "The only underused four letter word is L-O-V-E."

As a young girl I experienced "one big happy family" when my father held my hand as we marched and sang, "God is love and he who believes in love believes in me and I in him." In a period of deep depression as I slogged away at my dissertation, I saw *For colored girls who have considered suicide when the rainbow is enough* (Shange, 1975) with my close friend

Miriam Klein. I laughed, cried and reconceived my visions when an African American woman shouted from the center of the stage, "i found God in myself/and i love her/i love her fiercely" (1975, p. 63). Years later, I explored common and distinctive experiences with Irish Catholic feminist community psychologists Heather Gridley and Libby Gawith of Australia and New Zealand, respectively (Mulvey, Gridley, & Gawith, 2001).

Conundrums and longings that drew me to community psychology persist and shift as political agendas converge with conservative interpretations of religion and science to attack local and global communities. But I take heart when I remember that challenging inner and outer conundrums helps me to reconceive and repair myself within communities and the communities within me. I cherish early experiences of beloved community from my family and our Irish Catholic Midwestern New York middle-class cultures as I continue to create the selves, families and communities that I want for me and for and with others. Many theories, practices, role models, mentors and kindred spirits have helped me to value myself alone through realizing that I do belong to larger families and communities. I believe that we can and must create communities large, loving and diverse enough to hold me, you and all of us . . . together.

NOTES

1. Unless otherwise noted, opening quotes are taken from poems by the author.
2. Italics indicate a shift in time followed by retrospective interpretations of experiences and how they influenced career choices and commitments.

REFERENCES

Blair, D'Ercole, O'Connor, Green, B., & Mulvey, A. (1978, August). The representation of women in community psychology. Paper presented at the American Psychological Association Annual Meetings, Toronto, Canada.

Day, D. (1952). *The long loneliness*. New York: Harper and Brothers.

Frost, R. (1979). Death of the hired man. In E. C. Lathem (Ed.), *The poetry of Robert Frost* (pp. 34-40). New York: Henry Holt and Company.

Kuhn, T. (1970). *The structure of scientific revolutions*. Chicago, IL: University of Chicago Press.

Leidig, M. W. (1977). Women in community psychology: A feminist perspective. In I. Iscoe, B. L. Bloom, & C. D. Spielberger (Eds.), *Community psychology in transition* (pp. 274-277). Washington, DC: Hemisphere Publishing.

Lorde, A. (1984). Poetry is not a luxury. In A. Lorde (Ed.), *Sister outsider* (pp. 36-39). Trumansburg, NY: Crossing Press.

Lorde, A. (1984). The transformation of silence into language and action. In A. Lorde (Ed.), *Sister outsider* (pp. 40-44). Trumansburg, NY: Crossing Press.
McCourt, F. (1996). *Angela's ashes*. New York: Scribner.
Mulvey, A. (1988). Community psychology and feminism: Tensions and commonalities. *Journal of Community Psychology, 16*(1), 70-83.
Mulvey, A., D'Ercole, A., & Blair, R. (Eds.) (1988). Women in the community [Special issue]. *Journal of Community Psychology, 16*(1).
Mulvey, A., Gridley, H., & Gawith, L. (2001). Convent girls, feminism and community psychology. *Journal of Community Psychology, 29*, 563-584.
Park Slope Food Coop (www.foodcoop.com/PSFC/retrieved 08/26/05).

doi:10.1300/J005v35n01_02

Psychology in the Community: A Community Psychologist Looks at 30 Years in Community Mental Health

John Morgan

Voices for Virginia's Children

SUMMARY. I review my 30 years in the community mental health field, emphasizing the personal and historical context that shaped this career. I especially highlight the origins of the values that guided significant career decisions, including family, neighborhood, religious and educational influences. The core guiding value was the belief that public service is both a privilege and an obligation, and that righting social injustice through such service is a noble calling. I trace the evolution of my thoughts and actions reflecting this value, from an early desire to "help children," through preparation to become a child psychologist, and ultimately to practice in a public community mental health setting and a career dedicated first to primary prevention and then to broader safety net services for those in need. I highlight a corresponding intellectual evolution as well, a progressive change in identity from "clinical psychologist in the community" to community psychologist. doi:10.1300/J005v35n01_03

Address correspondence to: John Morgan, Voices for Virginia's Children, 701 E. Franklin Street, Suite 807, Richmond, VA 23219.

[Haworth co-indexing entry note]: "Psychology in the Community: A Community Psychologist Looks at 30 Years in Community Mental Health." Morgan, John. Co-published simultaneously in *Journal of Prevention & Intervention in the Community* (The Haworth Press) Vol. 35, No. 1, 2008, pp. 29-43; and: *Community Psychology in Practice: An Oral History Through the Stories of Five Community Psychologists* (ed: James G. Kelly, and Anna V. Song) The Haworth Press, 2008, pp. 29-43. Single or multiple copies of this article are available for a fee from The Haworth Document Delivery Service [1-800-HAWORTH, 9:00 a.m. - 5:00 p.m. (EST). E-mail address: docdelivery@haworthpress.com].

Available online at http://jpic.haworthpress.com

doi:10.1300/J005v35n01_03

KEYWORDS. Biography of community psychologist, community psychologist in applied setting, motivations and inspirations for applied careers, community psychologist in public service

INTRODUCTION

I have been asked to describe my career as an applied community psychologist, and especially to reflect on the events, circumstances and people that influenced critical decisions along the way. For those of you who have written an autobiographical piece of your own, let me extend my admiration. For those who haven't, please note that the flattering aspects of being asked may be barely enough to propel you all the way through this humbling and self-conscious assignment. In the end it proves extremely gratifying, but you may have to take it on faith until then.

I will review my background first, highlighting influences that shaped my values and the decision to become a psychologist. Then I will sketch my career chronologically, before retracing that path to elaborate on the important contexts and influences that guided key decisions. I must confess that it was not my intention early on to become a community psychologist. It was only after starting my career in a community setting and learning that my interests fit comfortably within community psychology that I began to identify myself as such. And only then did my work become fully informed by and strengthened by a community psychology perspective.

BACKGROUND AND EARLY INFLUENCES

Family and Neighborhood

I was born in 1948 and grew up in Springfield, Massachusetts, the oldest of four brothers in a working class family. My neighborhood, Hungry Hill, was predominantly Irish Catholic, with a share of Italian, Polish, French-Canadian and other nationalities. I still find it remarkable that within a mile or so of my house I could attend Mass in any of six languages. My father's family was Canuck (Morgan may have been Moquin before they left Quebec). My grandmother's cousin was the famous Brother Andre, who is one step short of being canonized a saint for the cures he performed on pilgrims to his shrine in Montreal, now the landmark St. Joseph's Oratory. Those near-saintly connections were almost enough to fully legitimize my father in the eyes of Mom's family but not to fully redeem her for being the first Foley to marry outside her Irish tribe. Nevertheless it was a successful marriage with two achievements I can note here: they raised me in such a way that I never once doubted that they loved me; and they bore with great dignity and perseverance the many trials of raising my brother Joe, helping him to cope with his multiple disabilities.

I like to say our ancestors were in the fuel business–my mother's were peat cutters from the west of Ireland, my father's woodcutters from rural Quebec. My paternal grandfather was a bricklayer and stone mason. My mother's father emigrated from County Kerry just before World War I, and worked for the city utility department. My father was the salesman for a local oil and coal firm and later started his own electric heating supply business. My mother was not employed, nor were any of my friends' mothers. Among the adults in our neighborhood there was not a single college graduate. My family's circle of friends contained not a single non-Catholic, nor any Republicans.

Clearly this was an insular, almost tribal context for my development. Its strengths, however, have always seemed to me to far outweigh its disadvantages. The neighborhood's values were conventional, and we learned right from wrong, or at least the Catholic version, because it was universally reinforced throughout the neighborhood. It transmitted a strong sense of ethnic pride and identification and belonging, and paradoxically a great appreciation for ethnic diversity–though homogeneously Catholic, the neighborhood's different nationalities retained their unique cultural attributes and we grew up learning and respecting these differences.

Broader Horizons

Fortunately, two circumstances broadened this narrow perspective. One I will call political consciousness. I grew up constantly exposed to local ward-level politics, and many of our relatives, beneficiaries of Democratic party patronage, worked for the city. I was persuaded early on that government actually helped people, and that working for government was an honorable calling. (I learned later, of course, that this patronage system was inherently unfair and discriminatory.)

One other influence accelerated this political consciousness. I was 12 years old in 1960, the year John F. Kennedy ran for president. It is almost impossible 45 years later to convey the intensity of Irish Catholic pride and identity fostered by his election. I watched every minute of the coverage of the inauguration (the blizzard had closed schools), and I remember running to the kitchen to tell my mother about the Peace Corps and the "Ask not what your country can do for you" charge. I can still name every Kennedy cabinet secretary (I can't recall the names of today's, however). To say that JFK inspired me doesn't do justice to the effect his election had on my emerging social consciousness and idealism. Without knowing its exact shape, I already aspired to a career in public service, thinking of it even then as a noble calling.

The second broadening force was the local Boys Club, located in an adjoining poorer, mostly minority neighborhood. The only official membership requirement was the annual fee (my first year cost $3.00). The more challenging unofficial requirement was that you learn to play alongside Negroes! It was a fun and engaging place, fun enough to overcome our reluctance to associate with "colored kids." So we played and competed and sometimes fought, on an equal footing with black kids who became our friends. We clearly lived in separate, unequal worlds, but this exposure was a powerful real-world education in racial tolerance. Significantly, the emergence of the civil rights struggle in the South coincided with my coming-of-age at the Club. Temperamentally, I think I was wired to identify with anyone being victimized or treated unfairly–the only two fights I had growing up came while sticking up for someone who was being picked on (getting bloodied both times was incentive to develop non-violent approaches to defending the downtrodden). My parents also imparted a strong sense of fairness and justice, so I would have felt strongly anyway about what I saw on the news from Birmingham and Selma and elsewhere. The effect was greater because I knew black kids and something of their lives in the North End.

The Boys Club was formative in another way. During high school my friends and I had part-time jobs at the Club and summer jobs as camp counselors. They didn't pay us much, but we might have done it for free because it made us feel important and useful. And the experience touched me in a more fundamental way. The Club attracted mostly children from disadvantaged circumstances, and I found that I had the personal qualities to connect with young people. This boosted my self-confidence greatly, and satisfied my emerging idealism by providing a small way to address the social injustices I was just beginning to understand. From this experience, I knew early on my career would involve helping disadvantaged kids.

EARLY MENTOR

The Boys Club soon gave even more shape and direction to my notion of a public service career helping young people. The Club had very dedicated staff members, and one in particular became a mentor and friend. He was such a likeable and positive role model that I might have adopted whatever career he followed, but as you must have guessed, he was a clinical psychology graduate student, and before I finished high school I knew I was going to be one, too. Because he so obviously enjoyed his work and was so skilled at engaging young people, he provided a concrete and appealing example of one career that could fulfill my aspirations. Despite spelling "psychology" wrong on my application (the guidance counselor caught it in time), I got into the college of my choice–Holy Cross in Worcester, MA–the first in my family and one of the first in my neighborhood to attend college. If I had been as smart then as I thought I was, I might have better appreciated how much my parents sacrificed so I could attend a private school. Add that to their list of achievements.

College

Let me state the obvious first: yes, I became a psychology major and achieved an academic record that got me into a good clinical psychology graduate program, just as I had hoped. This path was pretty straightforward, so I have no startling influences or epiphanies to reveal here. Psychology courses were high-quality, taught with enthusiasm and rigor, so they provided both a solid intellectual base and further motivation to become a psychologist. My one setback (well, in addition to my first statistics course) was losing the election for Psi Chi president.

The college influences most prominent are not particular to psychology. One is simply the transforming personal impact of this environment-in-time. For someone from my background to be on a college campus in those years (1966-1970) was ultimately but very uncomfortably "liberalizing." Not that our small (2000 students) all-male, Jesuit enclave was "liberal," but for most of us, the struggle to find our intellectual and moral footing in the turmoil of that era was unsettling. I had friends who were enrolled in ROTC, and friends who defaced the ROTC building. I was forced to examine, then justify or modify all the knee-jerk judgments from my upbringing. This was healthy, yet unnerving, but led to more discerning and honest intellectual and moral reasoning.

Lastly, a comment on the obvious influence of religion at a Catholic college. My education strengthened my commitment to the Church's vision of social justice ("If you want peace, work for justice.") while paradoxically increasing my skepticism about many Church doctrines. The campus offered many opportunities for community service, and our required theology and philosophy courses buttressed these opportunities with a compelling intellectual and moral justification for such "service." I left college with a stronger-than-ever desire to make the world a better place through service to others. Though I now fall outside any conventional definition of "good Catholic," much of my thinking about service remains firmly rooted in a Catholic perspective. As I understand it, the moral imperative of this perspective is not just to perform charitable works, but also to reform the social and political institutions causing the conditions that harm people.

OUTLINE OF CAREER

I will sketch my career, including graduate school, mentioning briefly some of the influences that guided key choices along the way. Then I will retrace my steps and detail the themes and influences that propelled my career in the directions I have sketched.

Graduate School and Internship

I entered the clinical psychology program at Penn State in 1970, hoping to become a child clinical psychologist. The department, building a behavioral/cognitive behavioral specialty, had just added Ed Craighead, Al Kazdin and Mike Mahoney. My skeptical nature, honed by the Jesuits, pushed me toward approaches bolstered by empirical research, so their coursework and mentoring were influential in my adopting a cognitive-behavioral orientation. There were no community psychology courses, and no faculty identified as community psychologists. But at the time, my own perspective was not so much a "community psychology" one as a "psychology in the community" one. The only unease was a vague sense that, although being a clinical psychologist would be a good way to help kids, this would address only one child at a time and not broader conditions and influences. Ultimately I reconciled this tension, as we shall see.

Most of my classmates hoped for academic careers, while a few planned to be in private practice (we were all supported by U.S. Public Health Service fellowships, and I remember asking, but not out loud, "Do you really think the federal government is funding your graduate education in the hopes that you will start a private practice?"). I was the only one who seemed headed for a public sector applied career.

My internship was at a child inpatient setting–the Virginia Treatment Center for Children at the Medical College of Virginia in Richmond. The experience included outpatient work and a one-day-per-week out-placement at a juvenile group home. At this placement I had the autonomy to learn and practice consulting skills, which made it one of the most professionally significant activities of my early career. Another key feature was that my mentor, Al Finch, and a grad student, Phil Kendall, were conducting pioneering research in cognitive-behavior therapy with children. Participating in their efforts bolstered my cognitive-behavioral skills and led to several conference papers and one notorious deep sea fishing expedition. Another lasting benefit: I dated a young nurse there, and Janet eventually became my wife of now 30 years. And one final strength of the internship: the medical school gym was just around the corner, and I played lunch-time basketball almost every day. All in all, a slam dunk internship!

Early Career–Prevention Programs

I took my first job at a community mental health center in Pennsylvania, then a year later came back to Richmond to marry and begin work as a staff psychologist at a community mental health center affiliated with local government–the Chesterfield County Mental Health-Mental Retardation Department. Two events in my first year there had profound impact on my career. First, my boss went out on maternity leave, and I was asked to be Acting Director of Children's Services for that three months. I found this leadership role exhilarating. I don't think the temporary power went to my head, but I definitely felt "empowered" and knew then that leadership responsibility would be very satisfying. It was going to be difficult to leave it behind in 90 days and return to my line staff position. I never had to, however, because of a second event. The agency's application for a federal Community Mental Health Center Act construction grant was approved during this period, one stipulation being that we would have to develop Consultation and Education (C & E) services. I volunteered to develop these, and by then I had established enough credibility that my bosses agreed and also invited me to stay on the management team as "director" of this emerging program. This should be clear later, but for now I'll ask you to take it on faith that I couldn't have dreamed up a job better suited to my interests and values.

For the next dozen years, I created and managed a successful C & E program, which from the start I shaped to be prevention-oriented. This work moved on two tracks: one, searching out and installing research-based prevention innovations that fit the needs of our community; and two, reforming my own organization so that it could host and sustain these innovations over time. My staff (eventually five people) and I created and launched both universal and selective interventions in schools, pediatric practices, day care centers, Head Start and elsewhere.

Due to the success of these efforts locally, I had the opportunity to participate in state and national efforts to promote prevention services in community mental health settings. Virginia's mental health department was developing an infrastructure to support prevention, and I served as the first chair of its Prevention Advisory Council and co-authored the department's first comprehensive Prevention Plan. I was instrumental in conducting statewide training events that spread state-of-the-art prevention knowledge throughout the system. Nationally, I was invited to participate in efforts to promote prevention research and practice at NIMH, at the National Mental Health Association, and at the National Council of Community Mental Health Centers, where I served as president of its Prevention Division. These successes resulted in two national awards–the Distinguished Practice Award from Division 27 of APA (1990) and the Harry V. McNeill Award for Innovation in Mental Health from Division 27 and the American Psychological Foundation (1991).

Later Career–Behavioral Health Leadership/Management

Subsequently, I was promoted to a higher leadership position where for the next 15 years I managed our entire network of mental health and substance abuse programs. Here the tasks are system leadership and management of operations–trying to create and manage a seamless network of services, ensure high quality, build partnerships, and imbed the organization in the larger system and community.

MAJOR CAREER INFLUENCES

Let me return now to the start of graduate school–1970 (in the same month, coincidentally, that George Miller gave his "Giving Psychology Away" presidential address to APA). I entered with the ambition to become a child clinical psychologist, armed with a high degree of intellectual skepticism and soaring ideals about righting social injustice, strongly predisposed to a career in public service, and possessing not a clue about how all that could translate into a real job.

Public Health Paradigm Shift

One assignment during my second year, however, crystallized almost overnight my vision for this career. We were asked to write about career plans and how we would apply behavior therapy knowledge in that career. Unexpectedly, the research I undertook to prepare my answer changed my life. My search led to articles describing recent legislation creating a new setting for mental health practice–the Community Mental Health Centers Act. Conceived in the Kennedy administration and born in 1965 as a Johnson administration Great Society initiative, the Act established a federal program to construct and staff community-based mental health programs. It was rooted in principles of egalitarian social justice, outreach to unserved populations, universal access, local autonomy, and services in the community shaped to meet its unique needs. The values were compelling, but it was the act's conceptual foundation that I found even more persuasive. For the first time I read about a public health, population-based instead of clinical perspective on mental health issues, altering forever my paradigm for thinking about these issues. Coming to understand the fundamental concepts of incidence, prevalence, host, agent, and especially risk factors, health promotion and prevention was a profound intellectual experience.

This experience forged two organizing themes for the remainder of grad school and into my career. The first was a commitment to this new community mental health center "movement." It is difficult to convey here the early excitement and promise of this federal initiative. Its intentions went beyond treatment impact to embrace notions of the centers as community change agents, working to improve social conditions contributing to pathology. The movement's short history (from Johnson to Reagan, circa 1965 to 1980) belies the high principles and broad vision of the creators and their cause. I began organizing my learning around the notion that I would work in such a setting, and in such a way that I could impact not just individuals but the community as a whole. This reconciled my unease about the limited impact of a "clinical" career. Before leaving grad school, I had enlisted in the movement.

The second organizing theme is captured in George Miller's phrase mentioned earlier–"giving psychology away." The legislation mandates that centers provide Consultation and Education (C & E) services, designed to impact not patients directly but the various community agents and institutions which could in turn impact entire populations. C & E programs were to be the preventive arm of CMHCs, strengthening institutions and settings to render them less pathogenic and more health-promoting. Reading about C & E, for the first time I could articulate a concrete method of giving psychology away. Although I did not fully abandon the notion of helping kids via direct treatment, I now envisioned a career in which I would try to impact many kids indirectly via services to strengthen their "caretakers" (parents, teachers, youth leaders, clergy, physicians) and key developmental settings (schools, day care centers, after school programs, etc.). In short, I would become a C & E person. But I should note, too, that my thinking was still less derivative of community psychology than "psychology in the community." My hope was to translate clinical knowledge into community-based, prevention-oriented interventions, but clearly my foundation was clinical psychology, with a strong bias for behavioral approaches.

Consultation, Education and Prevention

My first job was at a small mental health agency not far from Penn State, which hired me to develop its first C & E programs. My tenure was short–my wife and I decided to settle near her family so a year later I was back in Virginia. But in that year I studied the emerging C & E literature and tested out how to apply clinical knowledge in this new way. The learning solidified the basis for my early career in two ways.

First, I was inspired by the work of the small cadre of pioneers developing C & E programs nationwide. Tom Wolff, Carolyn Swift, John Clabby, David Snow and especially Marshall Swift remain my C & E heroes. I became active in the C & E Division of the National Council of Community Mental Health Centers. My professional identity now was "C & E person."

Second, my thinking about how to do C & E took on a much more preventive slant after reading George Albee, Emory Cowen, Steve Goldston and others. It seems too trite or simplistic to claim that reading their articles was inspiring, but so it was. I began to think of C & E as the locus for public health-model primary prevention to reduce the incidence of mental health problems. I returned to Virginia in 1976 dedicated to C & E and ready to use it as a vehicle to pursue primary prevention in mental health.

Virginia was not quite so ready for me, however; there were only three federally funded mental health centers in the entire state, and no vacant C & E jobs. With some disappointment I took a position as a staff psychologist on the Children's Service at the previously mentioned local mental health program–the Chesterfield MH-MR Department. The agency had no C & E program or prevention activity. Yes, there is some irony here–I had exactly the job I started graduate school hoping to obtain, but I now thought of it with some C & E snobbery as "just a therapist" because it would not involve broader, prevention-oriented work. The bigger irony is that within six months I was afforded the unexpected opportunity to create the agency's C & E program, and the setting proved to be a near-perfect person-environment fit. For the next dozen years, the job and the setting matched my temperament, values and skills in a most satisfying way.

Primary Prevention: A Twelve-Year Field Trial in a Community Mental Health Setting

I began to develop prevention programs under the C & E banner, most of them directed to children and using my clinical psychology knowledge base as the starting point. Brief descriptions of the first four programs we launched will give you the flavor. The first was parent education/child behavior management training. We developed hands-on education programs for parents of toddlers, teaching skills for coping with child developmental struggles and behavior management challenges. We modified and successfully extended these programs to families where risk factors were more prevalent, including Head Start parents. Second, we created a first-of-its-kind Child Behavior Advice program in local pediatric practices, where parents referred by their pediatrician could get immediate, research-based child rearing guidance. Third, we implemented in collaboration with the school system the Rochester Social Problem Solving program, a preventive social-emotional development program that eventually involved all 2nd and 3rd graders in the county. And fourth, we developed a multi-faceted divorce adjustment program that combined social support and coping skills interventions to help parents and children deal with the stress of divorce.

The organization's commitment to prevention programs gradually increased, due in large part to their credibility and success. Less than a year into my tenure I was able to hire a second staff person, and then in progressive steps we built a staff of six, totaling almost 20% of the organization's direct service staff. This was an almost unprecedented level of prevention programming in a mental health setting. How did such an unusual prevention commitment come about?

I have described some factors in this success elsewhere (Morgan, 2000). In short, the efforts: had a solid conceptual base and rationale that could be described persuasively to key decision makers; were based on model programs with solid scientific evidence; targeted known risk factors prevalent in our community; were delivered in partnership with existing community institutions; and produced program evaluation results that documented improvements in targeted risk or protective factors.

But the broader external context, reflected especially in two developments, was also a major factor. Nationally, the Reagan-era "devolution" of federal responsibilities to state government meant the demise of federally funded CMHCs. As they became dependent on state and local funding, many were forced to downsize or eliminate programs that did not produce significant revenue, with C & E often the first to go. Yet conversely, NIMH was ramping up funding for prevention research, exemplified by the creation of six university-based Prevention Intervention Research Centers (PIRCs) that began producing empirically tested interventions. Perversely ironic is that their early results were disseminated during the exact period when some of the likeliest settings for real-world replication were disappearing. For me, however, this was a period of inspiration and excitement. At the PIRCs, Irwin Sandler, Rick Price, George Spivack and Myrna Shure, and Shep Kellam were testing and disseminating interventions that informed our work and fed our search for research-based programs.

Simultaneously, Virginia's mental health system was developing an infrastructure to support community-based prevention efforts, opposing the national trend. My local success led to leadership in these state-level efforts. The relationships forged with others around the state during these efforts were among the most professionally and personally rewarding of my career, and our successes were among my most satisfying professional achievements. In particular, we built a cadre of highly informed prevention staff throughout the community mental health system, totaling some 100 or more staff qualified to implement the ready-for-replication innovations produced by the researchers at the PIRCs and elsewhere. This knowledge transfer enterprise was typified by two achievements. One was the publication of a manual providing systematic program design and delivery guidance to prevention staff throughout the system. The other was drawing national experts to Virginia on two occasions to train local staff. In the first, we held a three-day conference where most of the program researchers/developers listed in the famous APA publication "14 Ounces of Prevention" were the invited faculty. The other was the First Virginia Prevention Institute held at the College of William and Mary, with two dozen notable prevention researchers as faculty.

THE CLINICAL TO COMMUNITY TRANSFORMATION

Along with gradual program expansion came a progressive deepening of my understanding and appreciation of a community psychology perspective on the work. This was fostered especially by two events. The first was an invitation to teach a graduate community psychology seminar at Virginia Commonwealth University. So I, never having taken a community psychology class, taught one, first to myself and then to the dozen students. Preparing lectures forced me for the first time to systematically explore core community psychology concepts and research and to develop a fuller understanding of social-ecological perspectives. This solidified my emerging identification with the field and confirmed that I now thought of myself as a community psychologist.

Secondly, one aspect of Virginia's effort to support prevention was to foster ties between local prevention staff and prevention-oriented faculty at state universities. At what became known as the "Moton Conference," named for the rural (I almost said desolate) retreat location at which it was held, 20 or so faculty and a like number of practitioners were invited to explore ways to foster research-to-practice connections. There I met Dick Reppucci, who impressed me with his genuine desire to develop these linkages, and who in turn was impressed by the level and quality of applied prevention work in the state. Coincidentally, Dick was about to start his term as Division 27 president, and I am forever indebted to him for reaching out to me and urging me to become more active in the division. I did, and this involvement accelerated my community psychology development, and led to very gratifying professional activities as well, including service on the planning committees for the first two Biennial Conferences and the co-editorship (with Joe Galano) of *The Community Psychologist.*

So, after years of applying a mostly clinical knowledge base to primary prevention work, I was able to extend this work in ways more reflective of a community psychology orientation. In particular, my work began to incorporate social ecology concepts and attempt to alter institutions and social environments. For example, we worked to improve the development-enhancing characteristics of day care programs, altering the ecology as in the Perry Pre-school Project and other model "child-directed" early childhood programs. Similarly, we worked within the court system to alter the institutional practices that often added to the stress on divorcing couples. My work now more solidly reflected this new professional identity–community psychologist.

A COMMUNITY PSYCHOLOGIST IN MENTAL HEALTH MANAGEMENT

When my boss resigned, I took the opportunity to become the Clinical Director, responsible for leading/managing all of our mental health and substance abuse programs. I would be one step removed from the prevention programs, but in a position to continue to nurture and strengthen them. The real attraction of the position, however, was the chance to make good on the often unrealized promise of the community mental health center movement–to build and sustain a public-sector safety net of services that would reduce incidence and prevalence of mental health problems in our community; serve the poorest and hardest-to-reach effectively and with dignity; and promote community change. That may sound ridiculously noble or pretentious, especially in this age of managed care and the profit-driven mental health "industry." Yet our organization had the potential to pursue this vision, and the chance to lead this effort was also the chance to make good on my own core values and my original commitment to the "movement."

A complete account of this 15 years is beyond the scope of this paper, so I will highlight only briefly some broad aspects most tied to a community psychology perspective. Many of the most meaningful and principled innovations in community mental health today emanate from values and concepts fostered by community psychology. My job has provided the leverage to advance many of these concepts in our service system. For example, we have adopted a resiliency-oriented, strengths-based approach to treatment and rehabilitation. We have installed interventions such as supported housing and supported employment that promote full community integration of those with serious mental illness. We have fostered partnerships with those we serve to promote self-determination and involve them more fully in planning and developing their services. We have worked in conjunction with partners in the human service, education and criminal justice systems to ensure more dignified and appropriate treatment of those with mental health problems. And significantly, we have sustained our strong commitment to and leadership of primary prevention in mental health.

A community psychology conceptual framework guides many of these innovations and therefore much of my activity. This framework is indispensable to my understanding of the issues to be addressed, and central to the vision, values and goals I articulate to lead and persuade others. In this way, I may be more fully realizing a community psychology orientation than ever before.

CLOSING REFLECTIONS

I close by offering two observations. First, it is clear that my 15 years as Clinical Director put me in a position with more reach and leverage and impact on my organization and community. This work has been consonant with my values and ideals and original career motivation, and certainly has been remarkably meaningful and fulfilling. Yet, it falls short of the day-to-day excitement and engagement and fun of the "prevention years." Working as a prevention pioneer, alongside similarly committed colleagues in a common cause, in a setting that provided support and autonomy, gave me unparalleled professional and personal fulfillment. While I have no regrets about "moving up," I want to convey to you how precious are those occasions when person-environment fit is so ideal.

A second observation is about leadership. I have had the good if somewhat accidental fortune of being in a management/leadership position for most of my career. The power to articulate a vision, define goals, create and install innovations, and especially lead and inspire others was challenging and exhilarating. However, nothing in my graduate training prepared me to actually *be* a manager and leader. Being an expert in a content area may be a necessary but hardly sufficient condition for successful leadership in an applied setting. Learning to manage and lead is as essential as learning a particular body of knowledge. Community psychology served me well in both regards–and I remain proud and grateful to be a community psychologist.

REFERENCE

Morgan, J. R. (2000). Primary prevention: A ten-year field trial in a community mental health center. In J. Rappaport & E. Seidman (Eds.), *Handbook of Community Psychology*. New York: Plenum.

doi:10.1300/J005v35n01_03

To Be Different: The Challenge of Social-Community Psychology

Irma Serrano-García

University of Puerto Rico, Río Piedras Campus

SUMMARY. Summarizes the author's life and how differences contributed to her selection of community psychology and to various choices she has made to further her goals. Focuses on her context within a colonial setting and on the significance of being a woman in her particular environment. Shows how clarity and steadfastness to ideals linked to divergent skills and a collaborative and participatory ideology have bred change. Signifies students' contributions to the generation of new energy as well as new conceptualizations. Finally, stresses the importance of international and interdisciplinary collaborations to enrich both our lives and the discipline of community psychology. doi:10.1300/J005v35n01_04 *[Article copies available for a fee from The Haworth Document Delivery Service: 1-800-HAWORTH. E-mail address: <docdelivery@haworthpress.com> Website: <http://www.HaworthPress.com> © 2008 by The Haworth Press. All rights reserved.]*

KEYWORDS. Social-community psychology, Puerto Rico, difference

---

Address correspondence to: Irma Serrano-García, University of Puerto Rico, Department of Psychology, P.O. Box 23345, San Juan, Puerto Rico 00931-3345 (E-mail: iserranog@prtc.net).

[Haworth co-indexing entry note]: "To Be Different: The Challenge of Social-Community Psychology." Serrano-García, Irma. Co-published simultaneously in *Journal of Prevention & Intervention in the Community* (The Haworth Press) Vol. 35, No. 1, 2008, pp. 45-59; and: *Community Psychology in Practice: An Oral History Through the Stories of Five Community Psychologists* (ed: James G. Kelly, and Anna V. Song) The Haworth Press, 2008, pp. 45-59. Single or multiple copies of this article are available for a fee from The Haworth Document Delivery Service [1-800-HAWORTH 9:00 a.m. - 5:00 p.m. (EST). E-mail address: docdelivery@haworthpress.com].

Available online at http://jpic.haworthpress.com

doi:10.1300/J005v35n01_04

INTRODUCTION

In loving memory of Irma García Oller (1921-2005), who supported my differences even when she did not agree or understand them.

Differences can be both a blessing and a curse. They can be a blessing if one has characteristics, knowledge and skills which make one distinct, help one excel and which others admire. On the other hand, differences can be a curse if that which distinguishes us from others is considered a deficiency or an attribute which others demean or ignore. In this article, I will emphasize the role of differences in my professional development and in my choice of Community Psychology (CP). I tell this story so that others with similar ideals may consider this field for themselves after comparing my life context, struggles and successes with their own.

THE FIRST YEARS (1948-1963): CONTEXT AND FAMILY

I am Puerto Rican. I was born in 1948, in San Juan, the capital city. At the time, Puerto Rico had been under United States (U.S.) domination for 50 years.

Puerto Rico has always been a colony. Spaniards arrived in 1493 and remained until 1898. The Island was handed over to the U.S. as war booty after the Spanish-American War (Bea, 2005). That year Puerto Rico became a non-incorporated territory of the U.S. (Scarano, 1993). After a series of U.S. military governors, in 1940 the Popular Democratic Party (PDP) began to industrialize and modernize the Island. In 1947, as a result of the effort of various Puerto Rican political groups, a "new" political relationship was created: the Commonwealth of Puerto Rico.[1] Puerto Rico gained control over some of its internal policies but the U.S. Congress withheld control over most areas associated with national sovereignty (President's Task Force on Puerto Rico's Status, 2005). Since the U.S. takeover in 1898, various groups have actively promoted independence for Puerto Rico, while others have expressed interest in becoming a State of the U.S.

My parents were in their twenties when the industrialization effort and the Commonwealth were developed. Both were politically active in the PDP in the late 40s and early 50s, which were also my first 10 years. Political issues and campaigns, as well as government problems were part of our daily conversations. The PDP slogan "Bread, land and liberty" spoke to both social justice and political freedom, goals my parents supported.

When I was born, they were beginning their academic careers as professors at the University of Puerto Rico (UPR). My father taught law and my mother, public administration. They had been dirt poor in their childhood and had struggled through school and college as a means to achieve a better life. Although they were still struggling to make it on Assistant Professor salaries, it was clear to me then, as it is now, that education was a means to change. This belief was bolstered by their friends who were either academicians or government officials. During those years the UPR, the State university where my parents were employed, had the country's development as its guiding mission. This view of service from within university walls was inculcated in me early on.

In 1955, when I was seven, we moved to Boston, Massachusetts, for a year. My father was going to get an LLM at Harvard Law School and my mother was getting her MA at Boston University. That year, my second grade, I learned of the sacrifices necessary to get ahead, of another culture and, most importantly, I learned English. My mother said I hardly spoke for a few months and then started speaking English almost fluently. I do not remember this as a particularly difficult task.

Being able to speak English has been indispensable for my education and academic achievement. Its knowledge makes me different since, although English is a required course in every school in Puerto Rico from the first grade on, only a small percentage of the population is fluent and most people reject it (Millán, 1997).

When I returned to the Island, I began to really feel different in 6th grade. Up to that point, I was an average student. Around December I had to take a national placement exam. Surprisingly, I got the highest score on the Island. I did not anticipate or understand this result. Immediately, I experienced previously unknown pressures for academic success. I was placed in an "elite" group of 10 students with whom I spent my high school years in an extremely academically competitive environment. We skipped 9th grade and took undergraduate courses in our senior high school year. Because of similar exigencies and skills this group bonded and became my support group for five years. From that point on, striving to be academically successful, and in that manner being different, has been part of my every day.

MY UNDERGRADUATE YEARS (1964-1968)

With this background, I never considered any option other than to go to college and graduate school. It was expected of me, but it was also something I wanted to pursue. I graduated high school in 1964, and began my undergraduate studies at the UPR, Río Piedras Campus at 16, enrolled in second year courses.

The first year was very tough. I was taking courses with students that were two or three years my senior and my support group–the "elite"–was disbanded. Feeling isolated for the first time ever was complicated with trying to decide what to study. I had entered college to study medicine only to identify my disinterest in chemistry and math. Then, I was assigned a Freud primer. The compelling nature of Freud's arguments made me see the importance of understanding individual behavior to better grasp social issues. This was enough to move me into the study of psychology.

By the time I entered my second year, the economic growth of the 40s and 50s was starting to slow down and the PDP had abandoned independence as its political goal. Large sectors of the population had moved to the city or migrated to the U.S. A large middle class had developed. Statehood followers had increasingly grown and independence followers had been persecuted and almost stamped out (Scarano, 1993).

I started taking Social Science courses and, still feeling very lonely, found refuge in politics. I joined the Puerto Rican Independence Party (PIP). I was convinced that the PDP was no longer committed to social justice and liberty. Only the PIP offered me the possibility of pursuing these goals. Its university members also became my first support group in college; one of them eventually became my first husband. Thus, during my college years at UPR, I was a devoted student and a political activist. Both roles were supported by my parents and friends.

I worked arduously within the PIP. At the time, the Party was not registered, and this was required to participate in the 1968 elections. This goal meant traveling throughout the Island to campaign for my ideals; it also meant being scorned and ridiculed by most, since independence was, and still is, a minority option in Puerto Rico. I coped with this rejection because of the certainty of my ideas, and with the support of those who shared the experience. I also learned of the importance of ideology and stereotyping and how most people will reach conclusions about others with little or no information, led by emotions, in this case fear. The party's registration was completed and it participated in the elections. Success in this particular task also led to increased self-esteem and maintenance of my beliefs. It has also served as a guide for future community interventions–to sustain long-term goals one must achieve short-term success.

Another experience was of great importance during my college years. I was invited to participate in a project entitled *Campus Teams for Community Change* which was sponsored by the National Training Laboratories (NTL). This consisted of groups which were formed on various university campuses to achieve changes compatible with the NTL mission (NTL, 2005). This experience enhanced my skills in teamwork, verbal communitation, facilitation of workshops, and innovative teaching methods. It also generated new opportunities since I traveled alone for the first time to various cities in the U.S. and met people from different backgrounds. Again, I was different. This was an experience limited to few students and unknown to most at UPR.

As a result, during these years, I developed skills and values which were to accompany me all of my life: steadfastness to one's belief against odds, knowledge of what being in the minority entails, and the importance of organization, discipline, teamwork, loyalty and participatory decision-making.

TRANSITION: TEACHING AND COUNSELING (1968-1973)

Upon graduation from college in 1968, I applied to graduate school in Puerto Rico and received my MA in psychology at the same institution in 1970. Although at the time the MA at UPR was in General Psychology, I took all my electives in Social Psychology. My MA thesis focused on political attitudes. I wrote it in English because my advisor was a visiting professor from the U.S. His encouragement led me to present my results at the APA Convention in 1971, a "feat" which was also unheard of at the time for Puerto Rican students who studied on the Island.

While in graduate school at UPR, I became one of the founding members of a triumvirate of a women's group within the PIP. This brought to light feminist issues within the Party, a deeply *machista* organization, and confronted me with my first experiences with sexism. Up to this point I had not felt diminished or rejected because I was a woman. That it occurred in this group, created yet another experience in which I was different. As a result of our steadfastness and because we carved out a niche for ourselves that no one else in the Party could fill, we organized a sizeable group of women and eventually gained a spot on the Party's Executive Committee. This experience led me to understand the importance of gender in both conceptualizing and acting upon social issues.

While working on my MA thesis, I taught my first college class when I was twenty. I wanted my teaching style to fit my personality as well as to allow for student participation and creativity. Being essentially shy, I had to devise a way to teach that "liberated" me from lecturing but was effective in facilitating student learning. I believed that lecturing was a great way to transmit information, but not the best means to its internalization and application. So began the development of innovative materials and methods.

To this day, my teaching methods are different. I never lecture in my courses–well, maybe 15 minutes every once in a while. My classroom is a mix of workshop-like experiences, small group dynamics, and socratic question and answer periods. In accordance with the Freirian model (Freire, 1977)–within the established limits of an institution such as ours–students share in the responsibility of the learning process and in the execution of every class. Each student also designs his or her own evaluation process from a list of options (as many as 20) which I provide. When I began teaching, these methods were so different that students would line up outside my classroom to watch. Many years later, students tell me, with satisfaction, that the experiences in my classroom continue to be distinct.

For the next three years (1970-73), I worked as a Counselor in the School of Business Administration at UPR and taught a course on Human Relations in the Workplace. Two major learnings came from these experiences. On the one hand, I started to identify my mentoring skills while focusing on academic advising. The other learning was that I had to be willing to accept challenges like teaching a course for which I had no specific training as long as I had generalizable knowledge and skills. Mentoring and risk-taking proved to be essential later when I decided to study Community Psychology.

DOCTORAL STUDIES (1973-1978)

After five years of teaching part-time, in 1973, I decided to continue my studies. I moved with my husband and five-month-old daughter, Catrina, to Ann Arbor to pursue a PhD in social psychology at the University of Michigan. Again, the first year was tough. Not only did I undergo a personal crisis because of my daughter's illness and my divorce, the program did not fit my needs. It was too traditional focusing on small group dynamics and experimental social psychology. The interests that had driven me to pursue graduate studies–politics, social change, marginality–were nowhere to be found. So I started looking for options.

The first glimpse of a possibility was encountered in a course led by Richard Mann on group dynamics. Dr. Mann was not part of the mainstream of the Department. He focused on sensitivity training and group work which was on the fringes of traditional psychology. He had a group of students which I joined, thus creating a space for my interests. This was congruent with my continued involvement with NTL. For two of my five years at Michigan I participated in the Graduate Student Professional Development Program, an effort directed at developing professional trainers. This made me different again. I was not part of the "hard" psychology group which was housed at the Institute of Social Research and was not particularly interested in complex statistical analysis and research designs which were their everyday fare. I found support for my difference and goals in Dr. James S. Jackson who allowed for my divergent ideas.

After completing most of my required courses, I took an elective on Community Psychology with Dr. Cary Cherniss. This was 1975; the Austin Conference had just taken place. That course changed my life because I found a discipline, Community Psychology, which espoused most of the values in which I believed, but I had not yet seen within psychology (Bloom, 1973; Newbrough, 1973). These values also pointed me to new roles I could incorporate as a psychologist including intervening in community and social systems (Silverman, 1978). I focused my dissertation on creation of settings theory (Sarason, 1972) because it provided me with an opportunity to meld my group skills and social change goals. I completed my PhD with a joint degree in Social-Community Psychology, a mix which was uncommon at the time.

Ann Arbor, of course, was more than just school. I developed a core group of friends many of which last to this day. I also continued my political activism in those years. I participated in a student strike to increase graduate assistants' salaries. The strike was succesful, again strengthening my belief in the positive effects of organization and militancy to fight for what one believes.

I also experienced blatant racism for the first time. Blatant may seem a strong word for those of you in the U.S. who have experienced the atrocities of slavery and the discrimination and prejudice that follow. In Puerto Rico, racism is also ever present but has not expressed itself as brutally since slavery under Spanish rule. So, I will never forget walking into an ampitheatre for my statistics course to see all white students on one side and all the black (that's what they were called then) students on the other. Deciding where to sit meant identifying with one group or the other; I had never faced such a dilemma. The following years were a continuous struggle with this issue. I spent time with both groups and on many occasions served as the link between them. This experience allowed me to notice another of my differences: I could identify resources and positive aspects in most people thus facilitating their communication through me.

At the time, the University of Michigan had only nine Puerto Rican graduate students. They were in other Departments so it was hard to connect. This forced me to choose my friends among people from the

United States and other countries. Although I missed being with people who shared my roots, I learned more and influenced others by exchanging our differences. In some ways, I was living the community psychology values of cultural diversity and relativity.

THE RETURN (1978-1984)

During my last year of graduate school, I received a call offering me an Assistant Professor position at the UPR. I did not know that in 1975 the Department of Psychology had initiated a program in Social-Community Psychology and obtained a grant from NIMH to support training in Clinical and Social-Community Psychology (Bauermeister, Cintrón, & Rivera-Medina, 1977). They needed faculty to staff the program. In the intervening years, I had visited the island frequently and met Carlos I. Gorrín Peralta, a constitutional law professor, who was to become my second husband. This relationship, the job offer, and my interest in raising my daughter in Puerto Rico, spurred my return. So, I accelerated my dissertation process and by 1978 was back in Puerto Rico. There was never a doubt in my mind that I would return.

I found a Puerto Rico very similar to the one we struggle in today. Political parties reflect the different ideologies that have tried to support, modify, or alter Puerto Rico's political relation with the U.S. Commonwealth and statehood followers split approximately 95% of the vote, while independence supporters (PIP) account at best for only 5%.

Contradictions and situations inherent to Puerto Rico's colonial status for over 500 years, have led to pervasive social and economic problems, including alarming crime rates (Rivera Vargas, 2005) and mental illness (Ramos, 2000). Economically, things are even worse. Out of nearly 4 million people (U.S. Census Bureau, 2003), 48.2% live under the poverty line. Seventy percent of our industry is controlled by foreign interests (Hernández Colón, 1990). The manufacturing sector only created 187 jobs in the second trimester of 2002 while public debt skyrocketed (Banco Popular de Puerto Rico, 2003).

This is a bleak situation. Political, social and economic dependence as well as cultural imperialism characterize Puerto Rico's everyday reality. Although others may be discouraged by facts such as these, this situation has strengthened my commitment to contribute to psychology and change in Puerto Rico.

To reenter this colonial landscape was difficult. However, reentry was facilitated by the challenge of a newly developed and challenging program.

The Social-Community Graduate Program at the UPR was in its initial years. It was fertile ground for the creation of new courses and for the conceptualization and development of the practicum program.

One of the first challenges I faced in the program was the lack of practicum settings in communities. In order to place students in community work, I developed a project named Buen Consejo which applied various models I had learned from U.S. Community Psychology, in particular creation of settings (Sarason, 1972) and the educational pyramid (Seidman & Rappaport, 1974). The project achieved some change in the community and generated some highly skilled social-community psychologists who continue to be active in the field. It also generated methodological and conceptual innovations of participatory research which were extended to other efforts as well as theoretical frameworks linked to power (Irizarry & Serrano-García, 1979; Serrano-García & López-Sánchez, 1994). Participating in the development of the practicum program, and particularly in Buen Consejo, led me to become more involved in community organization and development. I worked in community settings for years at a time, not only contributing to citizens' empowerment but reflecting and theorizing on the process (Serrano-García & Rosario, 1992; Serrano-García & Bond, 1994).

The communities in which I worked also became training sites for undergraduate and graduate students. This occurred through practicum courses at both levels and generated student research as well. Again, I identified my passion and skill for mentoring and the satisfaction it generates.

During this time I participated actively in the conceptualization of our discipline. Our program developed a framework for the integration of Social and Community Psychology which melds a social-constructionist perspective with empowerment (Serrano-García, López, & Rivera-Medina, 1987). It has a strong influence of Latin American and European as well U.S. psychologists, sociologists and social workers (Fals-Borda, 2001; Krause, 2001; Montero, 2002; Sánchez, 2001; Wiesenfeld, 1997). It also includes a conceptualization of the research process where both intervention and research are simultaneous: intervention within research (Serrano-García, 1992). It is truly unique; another difference. With the exception of a similar program in Venezuela, our conceptual model is distinct, contextually situated and theoretically sound.

This process opened my eyes to Community Psychology in Latin America which was developing since the 70s with differences and similarities to the U.S. version (Montero, 1996). Without dwelling into the characteristics of both versions, I must stress that, ever since, I have been aware of the need to keep in touch with international contributions that are developing within our field. I decided then that I would publish mainly in Spanish not only because it is my language, but because it is also the language of the peoples I was, and am, committed to. I realized that U.S. Community Psychology, despite its proclaimed interest in cultural diversity and relativity, is really quite ethnocentric. I am continuously surprised when I attend different events in the U.S. and hear colleagues identifying gaps in the field which have already been attended to in other countries. For example, Latin America was way ahead of the U.S. in qualitative and participatory research, Freirian models, and community interventions. To fill similar gaps colleagues must travel and learn other languages so they may collaborate in projects and access literature published in other tongues.

My first formal venture into organized psychology also occurred in those years. Two events were particularly formative. The first was my participation in the Interamerican Congress of Psychology in Cuba in 1981 which nurtured my desire to continue collaborating and exchanging ideas with members of that organization. The second was my appointment to the Task Force of Psychology and Public Policy of the American Psychological Association (APA). Its goal was to recommend strategies to increase psychologists' participation in public policy processes. Not only did I learn a lot about public policy, I also carried out the first research project on the subject in Puerto Rico, and met Edward Seidman and N. Dickon Repucci. This friendship led me to become more active in Division 27 of APA (then the Division of Community Psychology).

These years were full of hard work, many satisfactions and some barriers. Barriers stemmed from Social-Community Psychology being a new discipline in search of identity and legitimacy within the University and the country, from a lack of resources and from the perception of others in the Department that we were radical and too political. In their view this could not lead to sound science. However, because of our success in defining our theoretical model and the visibility of our academic and community efforts, many of these barriers were overcome. By this time, it is clear that our work on social constructionism, empowerment and participatory research synthesized ideas of Latin American theorists and U.S. scholars generating a community psychology which was both a product of and a response to Puerto Rican and Latin American communities.

BACK TO SCHOOL (1984-1986)

As a result of my community experiences, I felt that a legal background would be useful for many of my community efforts. My participation at APA and my readings in Community Psychology also contributed to my decision to obtain a Post-Doctorate and then to study law. I obtained a Post-doc in Public Policy at Harvard Graduate School of Education in 1984-85 while my husband was getting his LLM and, upon returning to Puerto Rico, started law school. However, I found the legal educational process extremely adversative and authoritarian and decided to quit after one-and-a-half years. I did, however, reflect on the importance of interdisciplinary contributions and on the possibilities of working cross-disciplinarily. One did not have to know it all; one could collaborate with other professionals on similar issues.

BACK TO THE DEPARTMENT (1987 TO THE PRESENT)

In 1987, I was appointed Chair of the Psychology Department at the UPR. I initiated the implementation of the doctoral program, the first one in psychology in Puerto Rico. I conceptualized and sponsored two conferences on the Future of Psychology, one devoted to teaching and the other to the relationship between theory and practice. I also facilitated the curricular revision of the BA in psychology, fostered co-teaching efforts focusing on interdisciplinary training, and facilitated faculty's re-training in areas of their interest. Community psychology values such as participatory decision-making, social equity, the importance of evaluation, the importance of resources over deficits, were all essential to make my administrative role different from standard-issue administrators at our university.

In 1991, while still Department Chair, I turned my energies and skills to the fight against AIDS. Stimulated mainly by a close friend who had contracted the disease, I began consulting with community-based organizations and, as a result, an innovative project arose to train undergraduate students as peer trainers of youth in communities. The project was so successful that its participants were invited to provide consultation to similar programs in cities in the U.S.

I also created and directed the first post-doctoral program on AIDS Research at the College of Social Sciences at the UPR, sponsored by the National Institute of Allergies and Infectious Diseases. This program was a source of satisfaction and much conflict. Many colleagues within the Department thought that AIDS was a public health, not a psychological issue. It was also a source of frustration because the University lacked the infrastructure to meet NIAID's requirements for post-doctoral programs. Most surprisingly, my decision to publish in Spanish generated the consequences I had at times feared. One of the main reasons for rejecting the renewal of the proposal was that the PI–me–had few publications. Of course, the evaluating committee did not consider my publications in Latin American journals up to par with U.S. journals. They couldn't even read them. In a meeting at NIH a year after the proposal had been turned down, I was told that "English is the language of science." I wonder what Europeans, Asians, Africans and Latin Americans would think about that! NO, I don't wonder; I know.

I have been drifting away from AIDS work recently although I still work and train researchers in the AIDS field with a focus on gender and power relations. However, I disagree with the U.S. government's policy on AIDS (which is imposed on Puerto Rico) which focuses on secondary prevention and treatment, instead of primary prevention and promotion of health. So despite a strong institutional push for me to continue in the government's direction–because that is where the funding is–I have turned to other issues. I learned long ago to follow my convictions instead of my convenience.

AIDS work facilitated the integration of some of my interests, but it also distanced me from my more "traditional" community psychology work. Dr. Roderick Watts was a major force in refocusing my attention on the field when he asked me to co-author a Special Issue of the American Journal of Community Psychology (AJCP) on Psychology of Liberation (Watts & Serrano-García, 2003). That effort made me reexamine our discipline, both in the U.S. and other parts of the world, and rethink its emphasis. This work highlighted differences. Empowerment did no longer seem the vanguard of the discipline. An emphasis on liberation and a more interdisciplinary and international focus was called for.

Recently, I have returned to my interest in public policy. This focus is process oriented. My interest is in facilitating psychologists' involvement at this level in whatever their area of interest and expertise. Thus, I decided to replicate the study I had developed for the APA Task Force in 1983. The replication itself has yielded information which we have shared in different venues (Serrano-García, 2005). We have also received a grant from APA to initiate a continuing education course on the topic.

Throughout this process I continued my participation in organized psychology. Psychological organizations are essential to keep us vital, supported and to react collectively to issues of our concern. I have continued to be active in APA governance groups such as the Committees of Women in Psychology, Ethnic Minority Affairs, and International Relations. Division-wise I have been extremely active in the Society for Community Research and Action (SCRA) over which I presided from 1992-1993. I also represented the Society for the Psychological Study of Social Issues (SPSSI) on APA Council (2003-2006).

As a result of my commitment to Latin America, I became active in the Interamerican Society of Psychology (SIP). Initially, I coordinated the Community Psychology Task Force which for the past 15 years, under different leadership, has edited the community psychology papers at each Interamerican Congress in volumes which evidence the development of the discipline in the Americas. These are invaluable volumes written in Spanish, Portuguese and English; which all Community Psychologists should know. Besides this role I have been National Representative for Puerto Rico, Vice-President for Mexico, Central America and the Caribbean, the first female editor of the SIP Journal and President of the Interamerican Congress in 1995.

Throughout my career, students have always been on my mind. I thoroughly review their work and provide guidance for their goals and dreams. I am available at home, at the office, on the phone and by e-mail. Over the years I have supervised over 50 theses and dissertations. Students keep me on my toes. They are a source of vibrancy, challenge and they foster difference and risk-taking. Many of my students have become important researchers, teachers or community workers.

While undertaking these challenges I continue to receive support from my family–husband, daughter and father. Colleagues, community members, as well as students, motivate me to continue my work and aid me in generating new ideas. I believe that throughout the years my differences have inspired change and reflection, have allowed me to develop mechanisms to overcome pain and frustration, and have led me firmly along a consistent path. Overall, I see my work and my accomplishments as contributing, in the long run, to increasing diversity, to developing competent professionals, to improving the well-being of others and to the liberation of Puerto Rico.

NOTE

1. It is important to note that the official name of the Commonwealth in Spanish is *Estado Libre Asociado*–Free Associated State–which is in itself a source of contradiction as well as a manifestation of the subtlety with which domination can be sustained.

REFERENCES

Banco Popular de Puerto Rico (2003). *Economic progress* [On line]. Accessed February 6, 2003. www.bancopopular.com/popularine/pdf/prog2002_2.pdf

Bauermeister, J., Cintrón, C., & Rivera-Medina, E. (1977). Community psychology in Puerto Rico: Meeting the challenge of a rapidly changing society. In I. Iscoe, B. Bloom, & C. Spielberger (Eds.). *Community psychology in transition* (pp. 301-308). New York: Wiley.

Bea, K. (2005). *Political status of Puerto Rico: Background, options and issues in the 109th Congress.* Washington, DC: Congressional Research Services.

Bloom, B. (1973). The domain of community psychology. *American Journal of Community Psychology, 1*(1), 8-12.

Fals-Borda, O. (2001). Participatory (action) research in social theory: Origins and challenges. In P. Reason & H. Bradbury (Eds.). *Handbook of action research: Participatory inquiry and practice* (pp. 27-37). Thousand Oaks, CA: Sage.

Freire, P. (1977). *Pedagogía del oprimido* [Pedagogy of the oppressed]. Bogotá, Colombia: Siglo XXI.

Hernández Colón, R. (1990, 25 July). Mensaje del gobernmador el Día de la Constitución [Governor's message on Constitution Day], *El Nuevo Día*, 63-66.

Irizarry, A., & Serrano-García, I. (1979). Intervención en la investigación: Su aplicación al Barrio Buen Consejo de Río Piedras [Intervention within research: Its application to the Barrio Buen Consejo de Río Piedras]. *Boletín de AVEPSO, 2*(3), 6-21.

Krause, M. (2001). Haci una redefinición del concepto de comunidad; Cuatro ejes para el análisis crítico y una propuesta [Toward a redefinition of the concept of community: Four axes for critical analysis and a proposal]. *Revista de Psicología, X*(2), 49-60.

Millán, A. (1997, March 10). Retraso lingüístico [Linguistic delay]. *El Nuevo Día*, 8.

Montero, M. (Ed.) (2002). Theoretical and epistemological aspects in Community Psychology [Special Issue]. *American Journal of Community Psychology, 30*(4).

Montero, M. (1996). Community psychology in Latin America and the United States. *American Journal of Community Psychology, 24*(5), 589-606.

National Training Laboratories (NTL) (2005). *About the institute.* Accesed on October 14, 2005 at http://www.ntl.org/about.html

President's Task Force on Puerto Rico's Status (2005). *Report by the President's Task Force on Puerto Rico's status.* Washington, DC: The White House.

Ramos, J. (2000). Retrato dantesco de la salud mental en Puerto Rico [Dantesque portrait of mental health in Puerto Rico]. *Diálogo, 6.*

Rivera Vargas, D. (2005). *Se añaden cinco asesinatos a las estadísticas del crimen.* [Five murders are added to crime statistics] [On line]. Accessed July 20, 2005. www.endi.com

Sánchez, E. (2001). Psicología social-comunitaria: Repensando la disciplina desde la comunnidad [Social-community psychology: Rethinking the discipline from the community]. *Revista de Psicología, X*(2) [Special Issue, Yearbook of the Community Psychology Commission of the Interamerican Society of Psychology], 127-142.

Sarason, S. (1972). *The creation of settings and the future societies.* San Francisco, CA: Jossey Bass.

Scarano, F. (1993). *Puerto Rico: Cinco siglos de historia* [Puerto Rico: Five centuries of history]. México, DF, México: McGraw Hill.

Seidman, E., & Rappaport, J. (1974). The educational pyramid: A paradigm for research, training, and manpower utilization in community psychology. *American Journal of Community Psychology, 2*, 119-129.

Serrano-García, I. (Ed.) (2005). Psicología y política pública 20 años más después [Psychology and public policy: 20 years later]. Special Issue of the *Revista Puertorriqueña de Psicología, 16*, 149-297.

Serrano-García, I. (1992). Intervención en la investigación: Su desarrollo [Intervention within research: Its development]. In I. Serrano-García & W. Rosario Collazo (Eds.). *Contribuciones Puertorriqueñas a la Psicología Social Comunitaria* (pp. 211-282). Río Piedras, PR: Ed. Universitaria.

Serrano-García, I. (1984). The illusion of empowerment: Community development within a colonial context. In J. Rappaport, R. Hess, & C. Swift (Eds.). *Studies in empowerment: Steps toward understanding the psychological mechanisms in preventive interventions* (pp. 173-200). New York: The Haworth Press, Inc.

Serrano-García, I., & Alvarez, S. (1992). Análisis comparativo de modelos conceptuales de psicología de comunidad en Estados Unidos y América Latina (1960-1980) [Comparative analysis of conceptual models of community psychology in United States and Latin America (1960-1980)]. In I. Serrano García & W. Rosario Collazo (Eds.). *Contribuciones Puertorriqueñas a la Psicología Social Comunitaria* (pp. 19-74). Río Piedras, PR: Ed. Universitaria.

Serrano-García, I., & Bond, M. (Eds.) (1994). Empowering the silent ranks. Special Issue of the *American Journal of Community Psychology, 22*(4).

Serrano-García, I., & López-Sánchez, G. (1994). Una perspectiva diferente del poder y el cambio social para la psicología social-comunitaria [A different perspective of power and social change for Social-Community psychology]. In M. Montero (Compilator). *Psicología Social-Comunitaria* (pp. 167-210). Guadalajara, México: University of Guadalajara.

Serrano-García, I., López, M., & Rivera-Medina, E. (1987). Towards a social-community psychology. *Journal of Community Psychology, 15*(4), 431-446.

Serrano-García, I., & Rosario-Collazo, W. (Eds.) (1992). *Contribuciones puertorriqueñas a la Psicología Social-Comunitaria* [Puerto Rican contributions to Social-Community Psychology]. Río Piedras, PR: Editorial Universitaria.

Silverman, W. (1978). Role of the community psychologist. *Journal of Community Psychology, 6*(3), 207-216.

U.S. Census Bureau (2003). *Census data for Puerto Rico* [On line]. Accessed on February 4, 2003 at www.census.gov/census2000

Watts, R., & Serrano-García, I. (2003). Toward a community psychology of liberation. Special Issue of the *American Journal of Community Psychology, 31*.

Wiesenfeld, E. (Coord.) (1997). El horizonte de la transformación: Acción y reflexión desde la psicología social-comunitaria [The horizon of transformation: Action and reflection from within social-community psychology]. *AVEPSO* [Special Issue], 8.

doi:10.1300/J005v35n01_04

My Life as a Community Activist

Tom Wolff

Tom Wolff & Associaes

SUMMARY. The author recounts his life and how it led to a career as an activist community psychology practitioner with a focus on issues of social justice. He tells of his upbringing, family and education as the background to a series of positions in various systems. The story shows an evolution from working with individuals to working with whole communities; and from working on issues of remediation and treatment to working on prevention and finally empowerment, social change, and social justice. The story of his life parallels the social issues of the time. Throughout the accounting of his life the author raises the questions that he was struggling with. The sequence of those questions is as follows:

Can I emerge as a community leader?
What do I do with that leadership?
Can my work in psychology have any relationship to the larger social issues?
Can my politics, social action and beliefs in social justice, be integrated with my mental health job?
Can I find a setting that will tolerate and permit me to do work to create social change and reduce oppression?
Can we build competent helping systems with partners from many sectors?
Can we mobilize whole communities around community crises?

Tom Wolff, PhD, is President, Tom Wolff & Associtcs, 24 South Prospect Street, Amherst, MA 01002.

[Haworth co-indexing entry note]: "My Life as a Community Activist." Wolff, Tom. Co-published simultaneously in *Journal of Prevention & Intervention in the Community* (The Haworth Press) Vol. 35, No. 1, 2008, pp. 61-80; and: *Community Psychology in Practice: An Oral History Through the Stories of Five Community Psychologists* (ed: James G. Kelly, and Anna V. Song) The Haworth Press, 2008, pp. 61-80. Single or multiple copies of this article are available for a fee from The Haworth Document Delivery Service [1-800-HAWORTH, 9:00 a.m. - 5:00 p.m. (EST). E-mail address: docdelivery@haworthpress.com].

Available online at http://jpic.haworthpress.com

doi:10.1300/J005v35n01_05

Can we use coalition building to make a difference in quality of life? And finally: How can our spirituality inform our work for social change and how can our social change work to inform our spirituality? doi:10.1300/J005v35n01_05 *[Article copies available for a fee from The Haworth Document Delivery Service: 1-800-HAWORTH. E-mail address: <docdelivery@haworthpress.com> Website: <http://www.HaworthPress.com>*

KEYWORDS. Community coalition building, community activism, social justice and community psychology, spirituality and community psychology

INTRODUCTION

I live in a small town in Massachusetts. Leverett's government centers around the annual spring town meeting. The meeting runs all day and every resident who shows up gets to vote. We elect our town officials, pass our annual budget, and handle policy changes in zoning and planning. This process represents American democracy at its most basic and obvious level.

In 2004, the Planning Board brought a zoning change proposal to town meeting. It aimed at greater flexibility in land use which led to a clear sense of unhappiness from some residents. However, it also led to active discussion regarding the need for affordable housing. People lamented the loss of the economic mix that made up the town only 20 years earlier. The group agreed to form a new affordable housing committee. I knew I was hooked. At the end of the meeting, I gave my name to the Select Board as a volunteer for the new committee.

In this familiar action, I found myself stepping up to be a community activist. A combination of three variables usually pulls me into engagement: personal concern, positive social change, and the chance to make a difference. I care about the issue of affordable housing in my home town, the topic is tied to issues of social justice, and I believed I could make a difference. I knew the project would require an enormous amount of work, and it would take many years. All of these things are turning out to be true.

I'd already been on this path in my town a few times in the past. A decade before, at another town meeting, I had agreed to be nominated for the school committee. Passion about what was happening at my daughter's junior high school spurred me on. I spent three years trying to understand, manage, and effect change at the local elementary school and the regional junior and senior high schools. I made the decision to do this work in a moment of passion concerning an issue that involved quality of life for our community. Once again, I felt I could make a difference.

The most satisfying accomplishment of my local community building involved leading Leverett's effort to build a community playground at the elementary school. We recruited a wonderful planning committee, received donations for most of the materials, and coordinated the construction of a magnificent playground over three days of work. More than 100 men, women and children pitched in. It was an inspiring process.

These anecdotes illustrate some of what I've learned about myself and what sets off my activist spirit. The forces that have made me a community activist developed over six decades and have directed both my personal and my professional life. Each time the challenge appears, I've ended up in a fascinating situation, doing what feels like meaningful work. Sometimes I've succeeded, and sometimes I've failed.

I've also learned that every time I give in to the desire to get involved with community, I will face brand new questions about community life and about myself.

So I'd like to tell the story of my life of community-building chronologically, while highlighting the questions that I was struggling with along the way. My present work, which focuses on collaborative solutions, is the culmination of this lifetime of questions and experiences.

SEEDS

I was born in 1944 in the borough of Queens in New York City, the middle of three sons in a German Jewish immigrant family that fled Nazi Germany in 1938. Our community of Kew Gardens contained many similar Holocaust-surviving families. The dramatic family flight from Nazi Germany played a role in my social activism, although indirectly. My family almost never talked about the Holocaust or Germany. Over time I came to understand the Holocaust as the experience that brought my family to America and made them who they were. My father arrived with almost nothing in his pockets and built a successful office-equipment business in Manhattan. My mother painted abstract art while raising a family. As a middle child, I learned skills later useful in community mediation. My brothers and I played sports, collected baseball cards, and eagerly anticipated summer camp in New Hampshire. At camp, the sense of being part of an organized, thoughtful, funny, and caring community set me up for life. The country location began my lifelong passion for rural living.

My elementary school and junior high school were relatively small. However, any illusion of community disappeared when I attended Forest Hills High School, with 1500 in my class. The school was huge, the social pressures enormous and I was very young (graduated at age 16). I was lost.

Clark University

No surprise: when it came time for college, I found a small, liberal arts school outside of New York City. At Clark University from 1960-64, I found my voice, my interests, and began to experiment with community leadership and activism.

I was not initially involved with matters of social justice and social change. I became class president, and found I could initiate ideas and be heard. Clark had a great sense of community both among the students and between the students, faculty, and administration. The environment encouraged thinking, discussion, and critical exchange. I didn't know how rare that was in higher education.

In my senior year, I made a significant shift: from majoring in biology to psychology. The psychology department was alive, vibrant and challenging. Clinical psychology looked like a good match for my emerging interests. I began to know that I needed to work directly with people, not in a lab.

I grew more in the four years at Clark than in any similar period in my life, but only now do I see how formative my experiences were. The first unspoken question during those years was: ***Can I emerge as a community leader?*** Once the answer was clearly yes, the next questions were: ***What do I do with that leadership? How do I make it valuable to myself, my community, and the world at large?*** These questions were emerging as I graduated.

Rochester

I was accepted into the clinical psychology program at the University of Rochester, a high-quality graduate program where I had only eight fellow classmates.

Graduate school was a shock. Immersed in rote learning, I found myself without the intellectual atmosphere and stimulation I had become used to.

In my first year I was ready to drop out. But by year two, things began to look up. Academic classes were limited to Monday and Friday, while we spent the rest of the week in clinical placements. Looking back, I am amazed at the efficiency of our training program. At the end of four years, most of us graduated with finished dissertations and completed internships. I believe we were at least as well-educated as the current crop of

Ph.D. clinical psychologists who take five to seven years to finish and then begin internships. My dissertation was on the preventive role of group discussions in dorms, led by professionals and lay facilitators.

The next question about community activism that emerged for me was this: ***How can I use both my leadership skills and my growing knowledge of psychology for the greater good of society?***

While in Rochester, I began to explore the social justice aspects of community activism. I did some work in the African American community, during which I met with members of FIGHT, an organization created by Saul Alinsky. Opposition to the Vietnam War also became a focus for me. One Sunday I went to a Unitarian church to hear Allard Lowenstein speak about Eugene McCarthy's presidential bid. I became involved in McCarthy's campaign. In our little farmhouse outside of Rochester, where we set up a local headquarters for McCarthy, a rock was thrown through our window.

Meanwhile, in the graduate program we were being trained in one-to-one, remedial, pathology-based work. Yet there was a hint that clinical psychology could be connected to community change. Emory Cowen was introducing concepts of community mental health. These ideas sparked another question: ***Can my work in psychology have any relationship to the larger social issues of race and poverty and injustice?*** We heard Saul Cooper, a leader in community mental health practice from the Washtenaw Community Mental Health Center in Michigan, talk about his preventive work in schools. We read Reisman, Cohen and Pearl's *Mental Health of the Poor* (1963). We heard about work being done by psychologists in inner cities.

I left Rochester in 1968. Thrilled to be out of graduate school, I knew I did not want an academic career in psychology and a life in research. I knew that I wanted to work with people in communities on issues of social change and social justice. I was fascinated to take these concepts to another campus setting in a real job.

CLEVELAND

Jobs in student mental health were not plentiful. I found one at the Case Western Reserve University Medical School's Department of Psychiatry in Cleveland. I left for Cleveland with some trepidation. CWRU's Psychiatry Department was extremely conservative, and included a Psychoanalytic Institute–a rare combination. I would divide my time between an inpatient unit and the Student Health Service.

I saw that I could make a contribution by encouraging the use of social milieu therapy (on the inpatient units) and group psychotherapy. Getting a conservative Psychiatry Department to accept group psychotherapy was a terrific learning experience for me. My efforts met with both great resistance and wonderful support. I found it harder to move from my clinical work in student mental health out into the campus community. Neither the student health service nor the deans liked that idea.

So I sought other avenues for my community activism. We were deep into the racial disruptions of the late '60s and '70s, along with a more active antiwar movement. Urban communities like Cleveland were fermenting.

Two research psychologists holed up in the basement of the Psychiatry Department recruited me for a number of community political activities. One was the Save Ahmed Evans committee. Ahmed Evans had been accused of single-handedly causing the race riots in Cleveland and been imprisoned. Much evidence seemed to indicate that he had been framed. The people working for his release were generally older than me, and well embedded in Cleveland's liberal and radical politics. During a press conference, the group was looking for a fresh new face to represent it, so I was chosen as spokesperson. Interestingly, when I filed a Freedom of Information Act request with the FBI many years later, that event sat in my file.

Cleveland was not far from Kent State. When the National Guard killed students during an antiwar protest on that campus, the Case Western campus exploded. Students protesting the war sat down in the middle of the main street. The Cleveland police rode in on horseback, equipped with riot gear. The liberal dean of the college tried to negotiate between the two groups until the police decided to scatter the students. As I stood on the lawn of the student health service watching this violence, I had a growing sense of wanting to do more to end the war and to fight injustice.

In Cleveland, I met my beloved Peggy and we got married. Peggy is a remarkable woman and partner. Her own activism on a wide range of issues (holistic nursing, environmental illness, etc.) has allowed her to be patient and supportive of my many social change adventures. She has also taught me to see and value the pursuit of spiritual perspectives in our lives together. Our over 30 years of marriage have been magical.

My new question was this: ***Can my politics, social action, and beliefs in social justice be integrated with my mental health job?*** I was passionately drawn to the complex social problems that were facing our communities and our world. I felt helpless watching the United States lose over 50,000 lives in Vietnam. At the student health service, I was told that I could develop community prevention programs when the waiting lists for psychotherapy slowed down. This translated into "never." I needed to find a campus job where community work was in my contract. Peggy and I talked it over and we began to search.

AMHERST, MASSACHUSETTS

I found what looked like the ideal job at the University of Massachusetts Amherst in 1971. The student mental health service wanted someone who could combine counseling students with campus-based prevention and community mental health work.

Finally, I had the freedom to explore ways of developing effective community work. I began with more traditional forms of campus intervention: training peer counselors and paraprofessionals. In the next years, my programming expanded. We added preventive counseling to the contraceptive clinic.

I began to think of my goal at UMass as working with student paraprofessionals to create systems change (Wolff, 1974). This work built on my classmate Julian Rappaport's work on empowerment (Rappaport, 1981).

In the spirit of the time, colleagues and I brought Saul Alinsky to the campus and I got to meet one of my heroes. Alinsky had noted, "What follows is for those who want to change the world from what it is to what they believe it should be" (Alinsky, 1971, p. 3). The visit was, in retrospect, amusing. We had Alinsky meet with student leaders, hoping that he would encourage their activism. Instead, Saul–in his inimitable manner–asked how many were paying their tuition. When only a few raised their hands, he said, "I really can't talk with you. Bring me your parents; they're the ones with the money and the power." We should have guessed that he would turn his provocative tactics on us and the students. Regardless, we did manage to have a conversation with him.

UMass, with 25,000 students, was its own community. I could begin to see a relationship between the students who were coming for counseling and the environmental stressors. In fact, in one project, we used the Moos environment scales (Moos and Gerst, 1974) to give feedback to the residential staff. The logic of a community approach to mental health and systems change became even clearer and more tangible to me.

For example, the university owned 185 apartment units for married students, clustered off campus. Although the university took major responsibility for providing services to undergraduates who lived in its dormitories, it took virtually no responsibility for the married students. This population was under a great deal of stress: often one parent was in graduate school, creating situations with little money, young children, etc. More than a hundred young children lived in these complexes with no playground and minimal child care services. We began the North Village Program for Families (Wolff and Levine, 1977), hiring local moms and dads as paraprofessionals. This led to an infant/toddler program in affiliation with an academic department; the development of a playground; and, a range of other community-building activities.

I was greatly influenced by the work of George Albee (Albee, 1983). George was one of the few community psychologists I met who actively included politics and social change in his commentary. He developed a wonderful primary prevention formula that he presented to Congress. He included oppression, racism, and social injustice as stressors in the formula. I began to integrate these concepts into my work and taught a class for student leaders on planned organizational change: how to go about social change on campus in a step-by-step manner. I developed the course in response to a need consistently expressed by student leaders, who asked for help in becoming more effective campus leaders. In the beginning, the course was mainly for dormitory leaders. For example, I worked with the head of a 23-story dorm to create a highly effective community agreement that residents would no longer throw bottles out of the upper windows–its success reflected a major change in quality of life.

The students found that simple organizational-development techniques, along with the readings from Alinsky and others, were very useful. In the last year the course was offered, the president of the Student Government enrolled to see if he could figure out how to unionize the students. The heads of the Everywomen's Center and the Black Student Action Center signed up to see how they could increase the budgets for their organizations. Yet the Student Health Service felt the course no longer met its objectives and canceled my work on it. They also offered me a one-year contract, the equivalent of probation. This was the beginning of a pattern that repeated with many of my employers: they loved the community goodwill that my work generated, but were unhappy with any resulting controversies. In this case, my colleagues across the campus protested to the Vice Chancellor. My contract was returned to the normal two-year range. But, it was time for me to leave. I had demonstrated having a power base outside of the health service. This made my superiors uncomfortable. Although I could stay, the situation would only get more difficult.

My job had offered me an amazing environment in which I could learn what was wrong with our traditional helping system and could see that alternative interventions could really make a difference. There was no question that the programs we developed had a greater impact on student mental health than simply providing one-to-one psychotherapy. ***My emerging questions: What was the full range of community change interventions that I could help implement? How powerful could more formal networking be in helping to create change? Can I find a setting, hopefully a mental health setting (I'm a psychologist, after all), that will tolerate my questions and permit me to do work that creates social change and reduces oppression?***

FRANKLIN HAMPSHIRE COMMUNITY MENTAL HEALTH CENTER

I responded to an ad for a job as Director of Consultation and Education at a new community mental health center. This was as close to an ideal job as I could imagine. Indeed, the center's director actively recruited me to apply.

I held this position at the Franklin Hampshire Community Mental Health Center for just short of five years (1977-82). Funded by grants, my job was based on a local needs assessment that set priority areas as child sexual assault, domestic violence, and issues regarding the elderly.

At the start each staff person went out and talked to anyone who had anything to do with these three issues. After three months, my staff knew a lot about these issues as they existed in our area. They had talked to everyone, and that was not the norm. People engaged in the same community issue often did not talk to each other.

Seymour Sarason from Yale came to consult with us; this was about the time that he wrote *The Challenge of the Resource Exchange Network* (Sarason and Lorentz, 1979). When he heard about our work, he said, "Just keep doing what you're doing." He suggested that playing the role of middleman, connecting the pieces and bringing the community together around issues, would be sufficient for us. His visit reinforced the networking function at the heart of our activities.

For better or worse, though, we were more ambitious. We began to create programming as well, with a focus on systems' change.

For example, we worked with our Area Agency on Aging to reposition them with a focus on empowerment and on the assets of the elderly (Gallant, Cohen, and Wolff, 1985). We also partnered with them to look at the natural helping networks of rural elders to support people as they age, as an alternative to the increasing use of nursing homes and formal services.

Domestic violence was just emerging as a community issue. We pushed for formal linking between the domestic violence shelters and the courts. We brought the police into the room with the shelter staff and the courts. We looked at the recidivism rate of women who came to the shelter, and then asked, "what could break the cycle of violence."

I was influenced by Alice Collins, social worker and author of the wonderful book *Natural Helping Networks* (Collins and Pancoast, 1976). We had her visit us to share her work on the powerful social support provided by a community's natural helpers. Alice suggested that if you spent some time wandering in any community, chatting with folks and asking who would they turn to for help with a given problem, you would emerge with a set of names that were nominated repeatedly. She suggested building respectful partnerships with these natural helpers. I have never forgotten her teachings.

The community mental health work raised a range of questions: ***How could we fund and value prevention programming in the U.S.? How powerful was coalition building as a tool for community change? How could we build competent helping systems that included partners from many sectors?***

National Outreach

I felt I had found my ultimate job. I had left the confines of a campus to engage larger communities. I loved these expanded opportunities. I connected with the National Council of Community Mental Health Centers (NCCMHC), and became a national-level leader in Consultation and Education. Carolyn Swift, Chair of the Council on Consultation, Education and Prevention at the NCCMHC, quickly became my mentor, colleague, and dear friend. I met Bill Berkowitz, who was also a Consultation and Education (C&E) director in Massachusetts at that time. Bill has remained one of my closest colleagues for 30 years.

As members of the Council on Prevention of the NCCMHC, we pushed hard for increased resources for prevention and consultation and education. We organized C&E directors across the country and lobbied the national group. Those were heady years, and we had a sense that we could really have an impact on large issues. I began to hope that the mental health system might become a force for larger social change.

That vision ended dramatically and with amazing speed. Ronald Reagan was elected President and moved to shrink the role of the federal government. He converted federal community mental health center grants to state community mental health block grants, which gave control of these dollars to state mental health systems. Up until then, community mental health was almost solely supported by federal money. The state system focused on state hospitals and the chronically mentally ill. With Reagan's shifts, all the C&E programs in Massachusetts disappeared in less than 18 months. Almost all that remained were remediation services for the chronically mentally ill.

This was one of many times when I saw a lot of hard work vanish as a result of political change. My job had evolved to include management of the outpatient clinics, with a focus on generating more revenue; I was spending less and less time on consultation, education and prevention. It was time to move on so I left the community mental health center.

My experience at the center reinforced the idea that I could be involved with meaningful work that involved issues of social change and social justice at both local and national levels. I had become even more attached to community collaboratives as a way of facilitating change. I could easily see myself moving out of the mental health arena and into community change, but I had no idea how that was going to happen. I was deeply disappointed to see the collapse of C&E and the community mental health systems that had such great potential.

Mayor's Task Force

One piece of my work at the community mental health center that was sustained for many years after I left was the Mayor's Task Force on Deinstitutionalization, formed in Northampton, Massachusetts to deal with community repercussions related to the deinstitutionalization of both a major state mental hospital and of a large VA hospital. This was a piece of work that I had literally stumbled into. One summer evening, I was asked to represent the mental health center in a meeting about the placement of two emergency service beds in downtown Northampton. Deinstitutionalization was a subject that was rubbing many people raw including the police, fire department, and the Mayor's office.

The meeting was chaotic. The police and fire department representatives raised serious concerns about safety issues tied to having mental health patients in beds in the downtown area, as did a City Councilor from the affected neighborhood. The Mayor listened. The Department of Mental Health responded to the questions by accusing the city of holding a stigma against the mentally ill. Then, the Mayor got angry. The environment in the room was filled with conflict and hostility. I used my best group process skills to identify the issues, the disagreements, and future directions. Although the group agreed to establish the two beds in the community, the Mayor announced that he would not tolerate this level of discord in his community. He said he was creating a Mayor's Task Force on Deinstitutionalization. Then, pointing at me, he said "And you, young man, will chair it!"

At first, there was a lot of conflict. Meetings got loud. The Mayor could be the chief hot head. But everyone sincerely desired what was best for the community. The groups in the room began to understand more about each other's worlds. Over time the sergeant from the police force and the director of the emergency mental health service program began to sit down on a weekly basis to discuss their caseloads which overlapped by 40%.

This was one of the most profound learning experiences of my career. It was the place where I really began to learn what it takes to forge collaborative solutions. I spent the next nine years (1981-90) discovering how people who were in total disagreement with each other could find productive ways to work together (Wolff, 1986, 1987).

I came away from this experience impressed with the power of the collaborative process and with an even greater respect and understanding for politicians and the political process. I had a passion in my heart to do more of this kind of work.

THE BALANCE OF COMMUNITY WORK AND CLINICAL PRACTICE

After I left the mental health center, I expanded my clinical practice and my consultation work. For most of my early career, I had maintained a clinical practice, which surprised many of my community colleagues. Doing long-term psychotherapy and community building seemed incompatible. I maintained both efforts because, first, I truly loved clinical work. It reminded me of how complex and slow change can be. It also reminds me of the importance of history. Too often our approaches to community development do not involve a deep understanding of a community's history. Finally, having a clinical practice was a good insurance policy for supporting my family between community jobs.

I left the mental health center with a promise to myself that I would try to avoid working for any one system. Instead I would maintain a consulting practice and at most a part-time position.

COMMUNITY COALITION-BUILDING

After I had been in that mode for several years, the phone rang. A colleague from the University of Massachusetts Medical School Area Health Education Center (AHEC) asked if I would do community-building work in two old mill towns in the North Quabbin section of Massachusetts. The area's combined population was 30,000. The recent dramatic closing of a major employer had thrown the community into turmoil. The once stable, although not thriving, community was now full of hungry families who could not make mortgage payments. My colleague asked me to work with an informal group that was getting together to address the issues.

This was a direct request for coalition-building. I was thrilled. I spent the summer of 1984 working with this informal group to plan a major community meeting for the fall. The group consisted of representatives from the chamber of commerce, mental health center, hospital, political groups, clergy, and others. The fall meeting would focus on helping the community name the issues and mobilize to seek solutions.

Our successful launch in the fall began what was then called the Athol Orange Health and Human Services Coalition. No one had any sense that we were at the start of a 20-year adventure. We thought this was a short-term intervention. But we were about to discover a great deal about each other and about this amazing process of building collaborative solutions.

In our first years, we started monthly meetings to exchange information and increase our capacity to advocate for the area. We then, with the support of our state representatives, successfully lobbied the state for dollars for a new program to provide information and referrals to families in need of services. Once this service was running, we became aware of significant family homelessness. We began an emergency shelter in the basement of a church that evolved into the first rural family homeless shelter in the western part of the state.

We continued this pattern for two decades. We engaged the community, identified an issue, and moved to solution. At the end of the first years, the coalition expanded beyond health and human services. It took a new name, the North Quabbin Community Coalition, and created new mechanisms for grassroots engagement.

I was especially pleased to be able to integrate community building, collaboration, and advocacy. The coalition-building now involved working with whole communities. I felt like my beliefs in an ecological model could now lead to significant and locally-led community change.

The North Quabbin success spawned a request for similar needs-assessments and coalition-building in North Adams in the western corner of the state and then, within another year, for work in the communities on the far end of Cape Cod.

I was grappling with a flurry of new questions: ***Can we mobilize a whole community around community crises? Can we flip a crisis***

around into a positive situation and use it to create a healthier community? Can coalition-building drive community change? Can we integrate advocacy and systems change into our work and still survive? Can coalition-building make a difference in quality of life, creating real change instead of just providing more clinical services?

After a few years of managing the three coalitions, it became clear that these highly successful programs might provide a model with wider application. The W. K. Kellogg Foundation granted funding to expand the model to other Massachusetts communities, to evaluate the process, and to disseminate our findings. The grant allowed us to create an office that we named AHEC Community Partners. Until then, I had worked out of my private clinical office as a consultant with almost no support; now I became an employee of the University of Massachusetts Medical School. With a leadership team of Bill Berkowitz and myself, support staff and equipment (a copy machine!), we became truly dangerous. We began a newsletter, "The Community Catalyst," which ultimately went to a national audience. We soon became a national resource on successful coalition-building. We translated what we learned into easy-to-understand tip sheets to help hundreds of communities across the country struggling with similar issues (Wolff, 1998).

I was curious to find out that many ideas and resources for the field of coalition-building were coming from a variety of sectors, including public policy, organizational development, public health, and international community development. This is when I first discovered the work of Arthur Himmelman (Himmelman, 2001), a political scientist with some of the best thinking on collaboration and social change. We drew from all these fields to strengthen our own work and to create an interdisciplinary and multisectoral model for spreading information about coalition-building.

While we worked, we had been struggling to define the true goal of coalition-building in difficult, poor, and disenfranchised communities. ***Were we trying to repair damage, or to build something more positive?*** The goal of the coalitions was to improve the quality of life for the entire community. We saw improved "quality of life" as having two components: a competent helping system and a mobilized and empowered citizenry.

As the work expanded, we stumbled upon the emerging literature on the concept of healthy communities coming out of the World Health Organization and the Ottawa Charter (1986). The charter spelled out the prerequisites of health: peace, education, food, shelter, equity, income, social justice, a stable ecosystem, and sustainable resources. This document set an individual's health in the context of social determinants and the larger environment. It provided a perfect model for integrating many of our aspirations for our communities (Wolff, 1995, 2003).

We formally launched Healthy Communities Massachusetts in 1994 and began a Healthy Communities Newsletter and the Healthy Communities Institute, that trained community teams in the basic skills of building healthy communities and then supported their work. With faculty from across the country, we provided training in community mobilization, strategic planning, evaluation, managing diversity and the basics of coalition building. We lobbied the state to adopt a healthy communities model.

One fascinating aspect of the coalition work was our engagement with local legislators. We started each local coalition with the support of the local legislator (it is fascinating to note that in the very Democratic state of Massachusetts, two out of three of our key legislators were Republicans). The legislators were key supporters of and advocates for our work and ultimately became the coalitions' key source of funding. They would insert what is known as "outside language" into the annual state budget to support the coalition work. This tedious process involved the House budget, the Senate budget, the conference committee, and finally often an override of the governor's veto. We would in turn honor them for bringing resources or policy change to our communities. Each January, we would have a fascinating meeting with the state senators and representatives from each of the three coalition regions. The commitment of these legislators to this process was much deeper than that of state agencies, because they were committed to improving the quality of life in specific communities.

Out of Left Field

In my last years at the UMass Medical School we took on a new challenge: helping to enroll the uninsured in Massachusetts in available health coverage programs. In all our coalition-building work, we had been impressed with people's need for medical and dental care and had worked to devise solutions to the problems caused by the lack of universal health care coverage.

This is exactly the kind of problem that lends itself to the pursuit of collaborative solutions: many parties have some piece of the potential answer. For five years, the Health Access Networks (HANs) in Massachusetts collaboratively pursued solutions to connecting the uninsured with help. We brought together those on the front lines who enrolled the uninsured, the state agencies that provided coverage, and a state advocacy group. AHEC Community Partners provided the glue, the facilitation, and the direction for the meetings (DeChiara, Unruh, Wolff, and Rosen, 2001).

Partly because of these forums, Massachusetts became one of the top states in the country for enrolling uninsured children. The question during this time was: ***Can we bring the coalition-building model into the belly of the beast?*** In this case, the beast was the Massachusetts' Medicaid system, which had one of the state's largest budgets and most complex bureaucracies.

In my last year at UMass Medical School, the HAN meetings took on the topic of outpatient mental health access. Outreach workers had noted that they did not know where to send people who had serious mental health problems and no insurance for outpatient care. So we held six meetings across the state and discovered what we had known all along: there was no coordinated outpatient mental health system. We documented the comments made at the meetings. This report was similar to many others we had released. However, this particular information set off the Commissioner of Mental Health, who let her ire loose on the Vice Chancellor of the Medical School, who then let loose on me.

After 18 years at UMass Medical School, I was given the choice of resigning with a severance package or being fired for acting against the best interests of the medical school. Since there were hundreds of thousands of dollars of state contracts with the Medical School (much of it from the Department of Mental Health) the Vice Chancellor was very concerned. He could not afford to lose their business. So I resigned, and in the process made sure that the community coalitions I had created could continue.

This report would not have been one that I would have predicted to cause this much trouble. While the work we did was political and often controversial, our goal was always to serve the best interests of the community and state. Many other projects ongoing at that time contained more obvious battles that could have been seen as trouble.

As Jim Kelly has written, risk-taking is a critical part of the work of the community psychologist: "risk-taking in this context refers to being an advocate for real causes and helping the community move beyond its present steady-state" (Kelly, 1971, p. 901).

When I left the community mental health center nearly two decades earlier, I had promised myself not to work full-time for any employer who could terminate my position for political reasons. Yet here I was again. Lured by the vitality of the work, the independence with which I worked, and the ongoing support, I had been caught off guard. The answer to my question about the belly of the beast: *Not yet.*

I have come to understand that life is an adventurous journey. Some turns that look like disasters lead to new and fascinating opportunities.

So I expanded my consulting business into my present work, under the name Tom Wolff and Associates. A highlight of my national consulting work has been many years of association with Linda Bowen and the Institute for Community Peace, a remarkable institution committed to supporting community-based approaches to preventing violence and promoting peace.

I synthesize what I've learned through 30 years of community activism as *collaborative solutions (*Collaborative Solutions Newsletter, www.tomwolff.com*)*, and I provide consultation on how to create collaborative solutions to people and programs across the country. This has been successful beyond my imagining, leading me to work with new partners in new settings. Being my own boss suits me just fine.

WRITING

At various times during my career I would begin to feel that I had something to share that could assist others who were struggling with the same issues. That is when I would sit down to write. As more and more requests for materials and training on coalition-building came in to our office we began to commit more time to developing dissemination materials. This included books such as *From the Ground Up: A Workbook on Coalition Building and Community Development* (1995) with Gillian Kaye, a highly skilled community organizer from New York City, and later *The Spirit of the Coalition* (2000) with Bill Berkowitz, and journal articles (Wolff, 2001). Writing was a way to share what we had learned about community-building in one community with others. This was why I wrote. There was never any pressure or rewards in my jobs for publications; I was, after all, a practitioner.

In 1996 I also began a long-term collaboration with my valued colleagues at the University of Kansas, Steve Fawcett, Vince Francisco and Jerry Schultz, and the contingent back in Massachusetts including Bill Berkowitz, Phil Rabinowitz and myself. Together we developed the Community Tool Box (CTB), a web-based resource on community development for people in communities around the world. The Tool Box was developed in response to the dire need for easily disseminated community-building material for those actively engagd in community work. We wondered whether we could try to meet that need through the emerging use of the Web. The mid-1900s was still early in the history of using the Web to disseminate information. Ten years later, the Community Tool Box (Schultz, Fawcett, Francisco, Wolff, Berkowitz, & Nagy, 2000) has over 6,000 pages and 250 sections of community development material that are free and downloadable. The CTB records over 2 million hits and has over 100,000 users per year. As someone who was initially quite skeptical about the potential of the Web to provide support, I have been impressed and humbled by this experience. The challenge to our CTB team has always been to find the best materials, and then translate them in such a way that people at various levels around the world find them useful.

FAMILY AS COMMUNITY

The other major theme in my life has been my role as father and partner in my family. Learning to live successfully as a couple with Peggy, and as a family with my amazing daughters, Rebecca and Emily, has been the most profound community-learning environment of my life. When in my coalition-building work I define collaboration as "enhancing the capacity of the other," I am talking about a truly unique form of exchange. I believe it is the kind of exchange that has been the implicit goal in our family's love for each other. My times with our family are always the highlights of any year.

THE SPIRITUAL DIMENSION

Gandhi stated "Be the change that you wish to create in the world." I have learned over the years that we must create collaborative processes that parallel and reflect the outcomes we hope to achieve. If we are seeking a community that respects its own diversity, we must use collaborative processes that model diversity and respect. If we want to create a caring and loving community, then our collaborative efforts must also be caring and loving.

This is the spiritual aspect of the work that we rarely talk about.

Over the past 10 years, my work has been strongly influenced by my emerging personal spiritual practice. My new questions became: ***How can our spirituality inform our work for social change? And, how can social change work inform our spirituality?*** I returned to my Jewish roots with the guidance of Rabbi Sheila Weinberg, who taught Judaism as a spiritual practice. And I became a student of Ellen Tadd, a teacher of spiritual meditation. Through this I began to understand my commitment to social change as part of my spiritual path on the earth. I also recognized that I was not alone in these pursuits. This profoundly changed my capacity to do the work clearly and effectively.

I am now guided by key phrases that keep me focused on the integration of spiritual principles and how to actualize a better world. When I am in touch with spiritual principles I am clearer about my appropriate responsibilities and my aspirations for the world.

> *We can dream of a better world and we can make it happen. It is not up to you to finish the work. Yet you are not free to avoid it.*
>
> (from ancient Jewish writings–Pirkot Avot)

REFERENCES

Albee, G. (1983). *Prevention of psychopathology.* United States Senate Testimony.

Alinsky, S. (1971). *Rules for radicals.* New York: Random House.

Berkowitz, B., & Wolff, T. (2000). *The spirit of the coalition.* Washington, DC: American Public Health Association.

Collins, A., & Pancoast, D. (1976). *Natural helping networks.* National Association of Social Workers, 1976.

DeChiara, M., Unruh, E., Wolff, T., & Rosen, A. (2001). *Outreach works: Strategies for expanding health access in communities.* Amherst, MA, AHEC Community Partners.

Gallant, R., Cohen, C., & Wolff, T. (1985). Change of older persons' image, impact on public policy result from Highland Valley empowerment plan. *Perspective on Aging,* Sept/Oct, 9-13.

Himmelman, A. (2001). On coalitions and the transformation of power relations: Collaborative betterment and collaborative empowerment. *American Journal of Community Psychology, 20,* 277-284.

Kaye, G., & Wolff, T. (Eds.) (1995). *From the ground up: A workbook on coalition building and community development.* Amherst, MA, AHEC Community Partners.

Kelly, J. (1971). Qualities for the community psychologist, *American Psychologist, 26,* 897–903.

Moos, R.H., & Gerst, M.S. (1974). *University residence environment scale.* Palo Alto, CA: Consulting Psychologist Press.

Rappaport, J. (1981). In praise of paradox: A social policy of empowerment over prevention. *American Journal of Community Psychology, 9,* 1-25.

Reisman, F., Cohen, J., & Pearl, A. (Eds.) (1963). *Mental health of the poor.* New York: The Free Press.

Sarason, S., & Lorentz, E. (1979). *The challenge of the Resource Exchange Network.* San Francisco: Jossey Bass.

Shultz, J., Fawcett, S., Francisco, V., Wolff, T., Berkowitz, B., & Nagy, G. (2000). The community tool box: Using the internet to support the work of community health and development. *Journal of Technology in Human Services, 17*(2/3), 193-216.

WHO (1986). Ottawa charter for health promotion. World Health Organization, Canadian Public Health Association, Health and Welfare Canada.

Wolff, T., & Levine, J. (1977). Peer intervention in a married student community. *Personnel and Guidance Journal*, April, 490-493.
Wolff, T. (1974). Helping students change the campus. *Personnel and Guidance Journal, 52*(8), 552-556
Wolff, T. (1986). The community and deinstitutionalization: A model for working with municipalities. *Journal of Community Psychology, 14*, 228-233.
Wolff, T. (1987). Community psychology and empowerment: An activist's insights. *American Journal of Community Psychology, 15*, 149-166.
Wolff, T. (1995). Healthy communities Massachusetts: One vision of civic democracy. *Municipal Advocate*, 22-24.
Wolff, T. (1998). Coalition building tip sheets–compilation. *Community Catalyst*, newsletter of AHEC Community Partners, 1992-1998.
Wolff, T. (2001). A practitioner's guide to successful coalitions. *American Journal of Community Psychology, 29*(2), 173-191.
Wolff, T. (2003). The healthy communities movement: A time for transformation. *National Civic Review, 92*, 95-113.

doi:10.1300/J005v35n01_05

Odyssey of a Community Psychologist Practitioner

Carolyn Swift

Lawrence, Kansas

SUMMARY. Carolyn Swift has pioneered new professional roles in unconventional settings, including a Midwestern city hall and an interactive TV network. Her career-long interest in the prevention of rape began when she learned of the sexual abuse of adolescent males in the city's jail, and projected the long-term implications of such abuse for reducing its incidence in future generations. She explored the use of QUBE, an experimental interactive TV network, as a platform for teaching prosocial behavior to children–a preliminary step in violence prevention. Empowering women and men in relationships was a theme throughout her career. Her life path reflects her challenge as an early feminist–to combine a devotion to family with a passion to build a more just world. doi:10.1300/J005v35n01_06

KEYWORDS. Community psychology as a career, commuting marriage, feminism, interactive television, sexual abuse, social change

---

Carolyn Swift was former Director, The Stone Center for Developmental Services and Studies, Wellesley College, Wellesley, MA.

Address correspondence to: 1102 Hilltop Drive, Lawrence, KS 66044.

[Haworth co-indexing entry note]: "Odyssey of a Community Psychologist Practitioner." Swift, Carolyn. Co-published simultaneously in *Journal of Prevention & Intervention in the Community* (The Haworth Press) Vol. 35, No. 1, 2008, pp. 81-96; and: *Community Psychology in Practice: An Oral History Through the Stories of Five Community Psychologists* (ed: James G. Kelly, and Anna V. Song) The Haworth Press, 2008, pp. 81-96. Single or multiple copies of this article are available for a fee from The Haworth Document Delivery Service [1-800-HAWORTH; 9:00 a.m. - 5:00 p.m. (EST). E-mail address: docdelivery@haworthpress.com].

Available online at http://jpic.haworthpress.com

doi:10.1300/J005v35n01_06

INTRODUCTION

You Never Step into the Same River Twice

–Heraclitus

In writing this memoir, I'm struck with what stories, what images, what dreams and ideas to share from a long life. For most of us I expect there's a spinning kaleidoscope of possibilities to choose from, filled with snapshots of those we love, of our communities, of ourselves–in the heights and depths of joy, anger, passion, sadness, meditation, and grief. I've frozen the kaleidoscope in different slices of space-time. Here's what came out this time.

Childhood

I was born in Topeka, the capitol of Kansas, the first year of the Great Depression–1931. I was a middle child, with an older brother, Tom, and a younger sister, Julia Ann–all under five years old. My mother, Frances Oliver–red-headed Irish "Toots" to her friends and family–was a secretary when she and Dad met. Once married she devoted herself to the traditional role–taking care of home and family. Her mother was German and her father Irish, both from immigrant families who came to this country in the 1880s. Her father held a seat in the Kansas House of Representatives. In our family mom was a peacemaker, a mediator, a calm presence. She laughed a lot and loved to have fun, whether sledding down winter-packed hills or doing the Charleston with Dad.

My father, Tom Oliver, was a civil engineer. He worked his entire civilian life for the state of Kansas as a bridge engineer. Dad's mother came from Scotland with her parents. His father, an orphan, was 12 years old when he crossed the ocean from Wales. He ended up in the coal fields of Kansas, working as a union organizer in the mines. My father's public service was interrupted by World War II. He enlisted as a lieutenant in the Navy, was sent to Europe for the Normandy invasion, and then to the Philippines when Germany surrendered. I missed him in his years abroad. In our home he was a poet, a lover of art, classical music and Dixieland jazz. *An image that sticks with me is the night we took him to the train station before he went overseas. We left him standing outside the station in his formal Navy blues and white officer's hat, beneath the halo of a street light, growing smaller and smaller as we drove away, vanishing entirely as we turned the corner. We didn't know if we would ever see him again. It turned out we did. He lived to be 83.*

In college as a ROTC scholar, my brother Tom left for his tour of duty as a pilot with the US Navy after graduating in 1953. He was within two months of discharge in 1956 when my parents called to say they'd received a telegram declaring him missing in action over the Mediterranean on a routine patrol. *It was a silent, moonlit night when my husband Bill and I traveled the 25 miles from our home in Lawrence, KS to my parents' home in Topeka.* The telegram that arrived three days later declared Tom officially dead. His death shattered our family. My mother's faith helped her come to peace with it. My father never really recovered.

My sister Julia Ann was a top student, and a popular class leader. When, in her senior year in college she fell in love with a man from Iran and decided to marry him, Dad disowned her. Mother stayed connected over the years. That family schism, occurring in the same year as our brother's death, bound Julia and me in a deep relationship of caring and support. Over the next 20 years we became each other's chief family-of-origin caretaker, fan, critic, and loved one despite living on separate continents.

As a child I always saw myself in a helping role. Early on, when I shared with my father the goal of being a doctor, he told me I could never do it because I was a woman. Later I overheard him tell a fellow engineer that women were applying for positions in his department and that he'd had to hire one, but he'd see to it she wouldn't stay long. His inability to overcome the conventions of his time–to accept the causes of civil rights and women's rights–was a stumblingblock to a more positive relationship. My father was a much loved but increasingly distant presence through my teens and later adulthood.

Education, Marriage and Family

My husband Bill and I met on a blind date in my first year at the University of Kansas (KU). After we both graduated in 1953 he joined the Marine Corps and left for Korea. I found a job as an editorial assistant in a market research firm in Chicago, designing and analyzing market research surveys. In 1955 Bill and I both returned to graduate school at KU and were married the next year. What was unique in Bill was his capacity to see and appreciate me for who I was. He was comfortable with us both having careers at a time when women were restricted by custom to being stay-at-home moms. There was no specialty in community psychology then. The field was still 10 years away from its birth at Swampscott.

I was pregnant with our first child (a daughter, Lynn) in 1957 when we both received our Masters degrees–mine in experimental psychology and his in chemical engineering. After Bill completed his doctorate in 1959 we moved to Ponca City, Oklahoma, where he was a Research Scientist with a major oil company. These were my nesting years. During this time we had two more children, Mary and George. There was hardly time to read the paper for the cooking, cleaning, bathing, walking, playing with, and putting-to-bed and getting-up with three small children, their father and a German Shepard dog. Late at night I served as an instructor for KU's Continuing Education Division, teaching philosophy courses by mail. Ten years elapsed between my M.A. degree and my return to graduate school.

For as long as I can remember I held the twin goals of family and career. It was never a choice; more a destiny. It went this way: I would get married, have three children, stay home to raise them till they were all in elementary school, then chart my career. Bill agreed. And that's how it turned out. Although I have no regrets and would do it again, going back to graduate school after 10 years was like learning to walk all over again. Colleagues from my Master's days had gone on to Ph.D.s and positions around the country. Think of it this way: If you were asked to give up 10 years from your career path during your 20s and 30s–assuming you went into it wide-eyed, realizing the gap such an extended leave would create for you later and the game of catch-up you'd have to play–you'd have to decide what would mean more to you and those you love in the long run. I knew the career cost would be high, but here again it really wasn't a choice. I had to take the 10-year leave. Lynn, Mary, and George would have paid a higher cost, I think, if I hadn't. And I'm still playing catch-up, not with my career, but with the family who did without me at times in my catch-up years. As a member of the "I want to have it all" generation of feminists, I had it all. There were costs in both arenas–career and family. Those I regret most are those that affected my family.

Soon enough Bill began to chafe in the corporate world. When he was offered a position at KU in 1961 we both welcomed the opportunity to return to Lawrence. When our last child entered first grade I went back to graduate school. Our return coincided with the turbulent world of the Sixties. That decade brought chaos to many university campuses and KU was no exception. We marched with many others in protests–against segregation, against the war–down the main street, holding Lynn by the hand, pushing Mary in her stroller, carrying George, and ignoring the police officers photographing the marchers.

EARLY CAREER: PREVENTION AT CITY HALL

Amidst this chaos I was no longer satisfied with studying and learning. I wanted to prevent the injustices occurring daily in our community and began to seek ways to do this. In 1971 Betty Gray, the director of a community mental health center in a nearby Midwestern city, offered me my first professional position. The mayor had asked her to fund someone to work in city hall with the courts, police department, and jail to develop programs for alcoholic offenders, truancy, and juvenile delinquency. She'd already offered the job in-house at the last staff meeting, and no one wanted it. The prospect blew me away! I was free to develop the position as I saw fit! Here was my opportunity to work for social change from an establishment base. "Community Psychology" was not on my drawing board, but in retrospect I was doing it.

My years in city hall were turbulent, exciting, disturbing, and profoundly rewarding. Each day brought large slices of real life from a cross-section of the most needy. Exposed to the poor, the uneducated, the abused and neglected, and those charged with crimes who filed through city hall daily, I was soon moved to dedicate my career to changing the systems that spewed out dysfunctional human beings. I'm grateful to my mentor, Betty Gray, who made this job possible and trusted me to make it work.

One of the most serious problems I found at city hall was the adolescent males, most of them African American, who'd been arrested for misdemeanors and jailed alongside adult males–including felons. Some of these teenage boys were being sexually assaulted behind bars. Working together with the leadership of the mayor, the Municipal Court, and the local chapter of the NAACP, I put together state and federal grants to create a residential diversion center for young offenders. Instead of doing jail time they lived at the center and worked, attended school or found jobs.

Seeing teenagers leave this program better prepared to deal with their world, rather than marked with a jail term and a record, reinforced for me the value of collaborative community relationships and their power to bring about change. This transformation of the jail system's practices for dealing with adolescent males convinced me that systems change was possible, and that working from within community agencies is an important part of the process.

MID-CAREER: PREVENTION AT THE NATIONAL LEVEL

Community Psychology Enters My Life

It was in the final year of my dissertation that I learned of a new field, community psychology–focused on prevention and systems change–from KU Psychology Professor James Stachowiak. He steered me to new books on the topic. I read them hungrily. Here now, in this new field, was my home. It not only defined what I wanted to do. It promised a community of people who, like me, wanted to change their worlds. After six years at city hall I was recalled to the mental health center to develop prevention programs. This move marked a major turning point in my career. My work as Director of Prevention Projects began to involve me in mental health and prevention arenas on a national scale.

In 1976 I helped create and became the first chair of the Council on Prevention of the National Council of Community Mental Health Centers (NCCMHC). It was here I met Tom Wolff, a valued mentor, colleague and friend with whom I've regularly collaborated over the years. Under my leadership the Prevention Council accomplished several initiatives: a position paper, *Affirming Differences/Celebrating Diversity*, task forces on minority mental health needs and environmental assessment,[1] policies to address the ethnic composition of CMHC boards of directors, and the provision of bi-lingual CMHC staff. This work introduced me to national issues and leaders in CMHC affairs. As a result of this work and my increasing participation in national conferences I became a member of the NIMH Staff College, where I met Jackie Gentry, now a friend, then Chief of NIMH's Mental Health Education Branch.

Sexual Assault: Exploring Prevention Possibilities

As a feminist I was active in events and organizations involving women's rights and services. The prevention of sexual assault was a major focus. As a founding board member of the Metropolitan Organization to Counter Sexual Assault, I trained police, health, and social service workers to identify and treat rape victims. This training and my awareness of the sexual victimization of youths in the local jail alerted me to a glaring gap in official recognition of a major victim population. A literature review yielded only two studies involving boy victims. The state of Kansas collected records of sexual abuse of girls but none of boys, because, I was told, "it doesn't happen to boys." Sexual victimization was a role reserved for women and girls.

Puzzled over this systemic blindness to male victimization, I informally interviewed police officers, teachers, and social service workers. They all told the same story. If a boy reported sexual abuse they told him to keep quiet about it or he'd be labeled "queer" and ostracized. These victims were not referred to counseling or advised to share their stories with parents or friends. They were left with no resources to integrate their experience. It occurred to me then that young boys who were victimized might act out the abuse later in their lives in an effort to understand and master what had happened to them–a similar finding is reported in the literature on child physical abuse.

I began to wonder if early intervention with sexually victimized boys might prevent them from reenacting their victimization later, thus ultimately reducing the incidence of sexual assaults (Swift, 1979). Since incidence data on boy victimization were lacking, the first priority was to educate professionals in reporting agencies on the risk status of boys and advocate for these cases to be entered in official records. Pursuing this issue, in the mid-1970s I received a grant from the National Institute of Mental Health's (NIMH) newly created National Center for the Prevention and Control of Rape (hereafter called the Rape Center) to alert and train police, medical, mental health, and child protective service workers in this Midwestern city to the reality of the sexual abuse of boys as well as girls, and to the preventive possibilities of interventions with this population.

At the completion of our program the agencies from both Missouri and Kansas routinely collected data on the sexual abuse of boys and referred them to local resources. This project was not a prevention program. Rather it was aimed at laying a foundation for one by making the sexual abuse of boys public and quantifying it. The challenge now was to find a way to build on this foundation with a prevention initiative. The Twenty-First century scandals of the sexual abuse of boys by Catholic clergy, and molestation in school sports venues, bring home the tragedy of society's blindness to these victims, and to the potential tragedy of successive generations of traumatized boys who may in turn traumatize others in an endless chain of victimization.

As a result of this work I was asked to serve on several Rape Center grant review committees. Here I met many strong women dedicated to preventing sexual victimization, among them Gloria Levin,[2] then the Rape Center Deputy Director. A community of women researchers was formed. But instead of a geographic community fixed in time and space, the community was one of women from across the country coming together to empower women to stop sexual victimization. It was an exciting time. We took part in a series of Rape Center initiatives–grant review committees, national rape prevention conferences, a rape prevention workshop, and appearances before federal and state congressional committees. Inevitably our work spilled over into our personal lives and many of us formed lasting attachments. It was my privilege to be a part of this beginning.

The complex problem of preventing rape and sexual abuse inevitably dominated our discussions. My strategies in this brainstorming included interventions to reduce sex role stereotyping, and to teach children pro-social behaviors and alternatives to violence in resolving conflict. The goal of the interventions was to counter the patriarchal culture that produces rapists, and ultimately to reduce the incidence of rape in future generations. These were strategies I later tried to implement and continued to explore throughout my career (Swift & Ryan, 1995). It wasn't clear then how to design or fund such interventions on the scale required for research reliability and validity.

In my personal life our children were entering their teen years. By this time each of the five of us was doing our own laundry, cleaning up the kitchen and preparing one family dinner a week (I did two; Sunday dinner was "on your own"). Aside from having to outlaw tuna casserole, it proved workable.[3]

Exploring a New-Age Prevention Frontier: QUBE Interactive Television

In 1978 I was intrigued to learn of a new technology that had immediate bearing on my work, and that ended up changing our lives in far-reaching ways. The technology was interactive TV, available then in only two places in the world, Japan, and Columbus, Ohio.[4] Warner Communications introduced QUBE as an experiment in 1977 at a cable test site in Columbus. It was to be a national network, turning TV viewing from a passive to an active experience. By pressing buttons on a hand-held console, viewers could take part in talk shows, play games, rate programs, or respond to surveys. None of this is amazing now in the 21st century but a quarter of a century ago it was revolutionary. In six seconds the QUBE system could "read out" the results and telecast them to viewers at home.

Since the immediate reinforcement of responses is a prerequisite for efficient learning, the significance of QUBE's two-way interactive capacity for teaching was enormous. It promised to teach mass audiences of children–across the demographics of class, ethnicity, race, and gender–pro-social behavior by "talking back" to their TV sets in the safety and convenience of their own homes (Swift, 1983). An additional feature was QUBE's capacity to narrowcast, to simultaneously telecast different shows into selected homes within the same community, thus simplifying the delivery of experimental and control treatments to viewers.

QUBE was an ideal base from which to telecast programs to teach children pro-social skills, alternatives to violence in resolving conflict, and the reduction of sex-role stereotyping as first steps in preventing sexual abuse. As a realist I knew I would probably never have the opportunity to work with QUBE. It was highly unlikely Warner officials would let a 46-year-old woman with no experience in TV conduct a research program on their test site, let alone hire her. Even if I managed to gain their cooperation, my home was in Kansas and the program I wanted to implement was in Columbus, Ohio. The risks in leaving my family were higher than I was willing to pay.

Two events–one personal and one professional–landed me in Columbus, Ohio, pursuing the QUBE project a little over a year later.

The personal event was the death of my sister Julia Ann and two of her four sons in a private plane accident in Tehran in 1978. *"Life changes fast. Life changes in the instant. You sit down to dinner and life as you know it ends"* (Didion, 2005, p. 3). *I have little memory of the months that followed Julia's death. I only know that gradually, confronting the reality of her death, my own mortality, the slimmest of fragile curtains separating the worlds between myself and my two air-crashed siblings, and the short space-time slices any of us have to complete our lives, a resolve took shape within me to go forward with my life, to live more largely–to risk in previously unacceptable ways to fulfill my dreams–to do it with Julia as my companion.*

Julia and I had agreed that when our children were in college we'd take a year off. The two of us would travel the world together. We'd co-write a play. We'd patent an invention. We'd explore the QUBE potential. Together we'd work on fulfilling our dreams. After her death I felt a strong mission to carry the QUBE dream forward. So it was that when the opportunity arose, I was ready to take the risk of leaving home to do it.

The professional event that led to QUBE was an invitation from the Rape Center to participate in the first national workshop on rape prevention research. Serendipitously, the workshop was held in Columbus, Ohio. Some 50 women from across the country came together to share their work and brainstorm next steps in rape prevention. Here I met many women who became good friends over the years, including Joyce Lazar,[5] then NIMH Chief of Social Sciences. Reuniting with colleagues led to the sharing of dream projects, and I shared mine. Friends there encouraged me to return to Columbus and pursue the dream.

Back home, Bill and I talked it over. Our children were all now in college. He said I'd stood by him throughout his career (he was a chaired professor) and now it was his turn to stand by me. I could go with his blessing. The last piece of the QUBE puzzle was "how to get there from here"–where *there* was working at Warner QUBE TV in Columbus, and *here* was working at a mental health center in a Midwestern city 700 miles from Columbus. What I had to offer were my skills as a community and clinical psychologist. The best strategy, I decided, was to find a position at a Columbus mental health center and integrate QUBE's interactive services into a broader set of the center's community prevention programs.

So it was that in 1979 I interviewed the Director of the Southwest Community Mental Health Center in Columbus, Jim Gibson. I briefed him on the QUBE project and proposed he employ me to set up a prevention unit in the center in which the QUBE project would be a part. He agreed. For the next three years my time was divided between the center and QUBE. My long-distance phone bill was my great indulgence: it was the lifeline to my support system–Bill, our children, and friends across the country. Living alone I spent late nights and weekends meeting grant deadlines for (non-QUBE) prevention programs for the mental health center, and developing the QUBE proposal. I built a prevention department for the center with a staff of 10 and a set of prevention action and research programs embedded within the center's community.

I am indebted to Jim Gilbert for believing in me.

Ultimately I submitted a grant for the QUBE project, *A Media Approach to the Prevention of Rape*. The review committee expressed interest and requested a site visit. I'd given up many things to make this dream come true. Fate had teased me by making it easy: Bill approved, our children were in college, I found a center that welcomed me, and a corporation that valued my skills. All the barriers were dropped. Except this final one. I was at a conference in San Francisco when I learned the grant had been rejected. I was shocked and numbed. My dream was a pipe dream after all.

LATE CAREER: EMPOWERING WOMEN

> *Now, looking back, lessons I learned from this experience, clichés though they are: Depression is not destiny. Down is not out. Tomorrow's another day.*

My tomorrow came after it was clear that my QUBE dream would not be realized.[6] I found myself in San Francisco once again, this time as faculty for one of a series of NIMH conferences on Mental Health Issues for Women. Jean Baker Miller, M.D., the Director of the Stone Center for Developmental Services and Studies[7] at Wellesley College, was also there. I learned she was resigning her position at the Stone Center. She encouraged me to apply. Bill and I talked it over, he supported my decision to apply, and I was ultimately selected for the position.

The Stone Center was the essence of a feminist prevention career. Its primary mission was to prevent mental illness. Dr. Miller herself was a major reason to be there; she stayed on as Scholar in Residence, becoming, in my late-life career, a significant mentor. Her ground-breaking theories on gender roles and relationships, her eminence in the field of psychiatric treatment of women and men, and her personal warmth and intense dedication to her work drew me and many other women scholars and activists to the center. George Albee, a mentor whose prevention philosophy had attracted me to the field (Swift, 1992), was already a member of the center's board of directors when I came. He provided sound counsel throughout my watch.

The work focused on an agenda Dr. Miller had developed for the center around what were known then as "women's issues," which are in reality societal issues consigned to the woman's ghetto. These issues, her approach to them, and the opportunity to join my voice with those of this strong community of women resonated deeply with me (Swift, 1986). The community here is worldwide. Dr. Miller's writings and those of other women connected with the Center are read in many countries. Stone Center conferences and workshops are beacons for women around the globe to gather together to advance the work.

Working at Wellesley College, with its traditions of women's leadership and excellence, is an empowering experience, both as a community psychologist, and as a woman. The theme of empowering both women and men runs through the Center's work and is a part of its programs. Finally, the center had a $2 million endowment, thanks to the generosity of its founders, Grace and Robert Stone and their daughters, Katherine Kaufmann and Linda Stone.

At Wellesley I found my role to be more supporting the work of others than developing my own. My contributions were modest. Although I initiated some prevention programs, as Director my energies were occupied more in administration. I was creative in building staff positions and programs, maintaining the energy and direction Dr. Miller had set, and augmenting the center's resources.

During these years I was also active in Div. 27/SCRA as Member-at-Large on the Executive Committee. Julian Rappaport was EC

President at this time. His enthusiasm for learning from others, his commitment to building a Community Psychology Division where all are welcome and encouraged to share in the leadership, his deep and genuine caring for his students moved and humbled me. Through these experiences and in co-editing a book on empowerment with him, he became a mentor (Rappaport, Swift, & Hess, 1984).

After five rewarding years my Wellesley position ended as a result of a brain aneurysm, a sudden attack that occurred with no warning.[8]

Throughout my 10-year commute my home-away-from-home served as a way-station on my children's journeys from college to the wider world. Occasionally one came to live with me for a few weeks or months. Mary rented an adjoining apartment in Wellesley during part of my recovery. My children were building increasingly independent lives. Now I was lonely despite the kindness of friends. I walked home from work daily, often at twilight or after. Coming around the corner of my block I saw lights turning on in living rooms and families going about their dinner preparations, laughing together at the table, watching TV together. As I approached my house my heart would sink as I looked up at the second floor apartment where I lived, totally dark and cold, where no one was waiting for me.

My health crisis had changed my quality of life. I missed the intimacy of family. I resigned almost two years after my aneurysm, and rejoined Bill in our Kansas home. Leonard Jason (1993), who suffered a years-long bout with illness, put it simply. "I needed to be with a family or community, as a buffer against stress and as a nurturing place . . . When I entered the home of a loving family, I immediately began feeling a lot better" (p. 67). Being home with Bill again I found the peace, the safety, and the caring that was a vital part of my recovery.

LATE-LATE CAREER

Since I left Wellesley I've been active in the field through appointments to boards, APA and SCRA committees, and various publications. My interests in sexual abuse (Swift, 1995; Swift & Ryan-Finn, 1995), and empowerment (Swift, 1992; Swift, Bond, & Serrano-García, 1999; Swift & Levin, 1987) have continued to occupy me. It was a pleasant surprise to be elected SCRA's/Div. 27's President in 2005. I'm the first senior citizen to hold the post, an honor I'm proud of–for myself of course, but more for other senior members who may be encouraged to be active once they see how much they can contribute, and how much their contributions are valued. My interests have also expanded to the art world. As a board member of the Albert Bloch Foundation, I've become involved in studying the life and times of this artist, and learning of his work through his widow, Anna, a friend here in Lawrence.

CODA

Bill and I have just celebrated our 50th wedding anniversary. Lynn is an assistant professor of French at a small university in Pennsylvania. Her daughter–our granddaughter, Kathleen, 15–is into Japanese anime and graphic novels. Mary, a linguist, is a researcher in the Computer Linguistics Department at the University of Rochester, NY. Her husband, Juergen Bohnemeyer, is an assistant professor of Linguistics at the University of Buffalo. Our son George spent 15 years in the computer software business. He's now in Argentina seeking an economical, politically-friendly environment in which to practice yoga and meditation. Julia's two surviving sons–Tom and Cyrus John and their families, her widowed husband, Cyrus Samii, and his wife, Shirine, remain integral parts of my life.

Reflecting on my career, I've spent a great part of my time in what Kelly (1999) calls boundary spanning–establishing relationships and exchanging resources with agencies in systems outside my own. For most if not all community psychologist practitioners, this is a primary career role. Here I'd like to share examples of outcomes of boundary spanning–risks, benefits, and lessons learned.

A major risk is the challenge boundary spanners face in balancing their identification with their home system and the outside system. Over time, as they bond with the new system's personnel and become familiar with the vocabulary and values of the new system, they begin to become more a part of it. Without a secure internal compass about their role, practitioners can lose their balance between the two systems and fail to perform their role as anticipated–that is, they can fail to bring about the agreed-upon exchange of resources between the two systems.

I'm reminded of a fresh Ph.D. who was placed by a community mental health center halftime in a high-tech corporation. His role was to be an objective presence in assisting staff with work-related problems and to conduct ongoing research. He soon made friends with workers in the new environment, then openly sided with them against management, and refused to conduct the research to which he had originally agreed. He was terminated. The high-tech site was embroiled in turmoil over this man's boundary confusions. The contract with the mental health center was dropped.

Although we could chalk up this young man's unprofessional behavior to his inexperience and naiveté perhaps, the matter of shifting identities in consulting roles can be a role-related hazard, as it was with him, or a benefit. When I left home to seek work with QUBE in Columbus, I built my entry into that system on gaining a position in a community mental health center in the same city, using their local prominence and good name as a resource. I laid out this strategy openly with my would-be employer at our first interview, as well as my plan to build a prevention unit within his mental health center during my time there. Jim Gibson knew why I had come and my record in the field. He hired me full-time as Director of Prevention with the understanding that I'd spend half my time consulting with QUBE. When QUBE personnel later offered me a full-time position and I accepted, both the center and QUBE had benefited by the resource exchange between our two systems. The center's prevention unit, which I'd begun, was subsequently headed and expanded by Helen Jackson, a state leader in the field and a friend. She came to the center from her distinguished service as Director of Prevention for the State of Ohio Department of Mental Health.

The lesson here is to be as transparent as you can about your goals as you work in new systems, the resources you mean to bring, and those you mean to take back to your home base. The letter of agreement or contract between the two systems should broadly outline the process and products of your efforts, but leave wiggle room for creativity and adaptability to emerging conditions. My "system switch" was a benefit for QUBE, and a benefit for the Southwest Community Mental Health Center as well.

System switching can be a win-win situation for the multiple systems involved. When I was teaching police, medical, mental health, and child protective service workers how to identify, report and refer sexually abused boys, two of the trainees (a man and a woman), both from the same state agency, came to me and asked for permission to use the course materials. They planned to teach the course in their satellite offices across their state. They'd already gotten permission and funding support from their agency to do so. Of course I gave them the materials and my blessing. They left the positions they had and took on new full-time roles–sharing what they had learned and the course resources with their statewide colleagues. By changing their roles within their own agency they adopted the new system as their own. Two systems–the community mental health center that sponsored the training, and the agency that adopted the training for their entire state–benefited from this resource exchange. Thus small-scale system change was accomplished–ending again in a win-win, if unplanned, outcome.

Community psychology practitioners are passionate about their mission–promoting the process of empowerment and the goal of prevention in human lives. It is humbling and immensely rewarding to have a part, however small, in changing a system for the better. Keys to effectiveness include being open to the possibilities around you, thinking and acting outside the box, creatively finding your way around obstacles and refusals, and developing strategies that are win-win. My counsel to newcomers: If you have a passion to change this world into a better one, it's worth your energy and time to try, it's worth the risks, it's worth a lifetime commitment.

Give the world the best you have, and it may never be enough;
Give the world the best you have anyway.

–Attributed to Mother Theresa

NOTES

1. This task force resulted in a book: Insel, P.M. (Ed.) (1980). *Environmental variables and the prevention of mental illness.* Lexington, MA: Lexington Books.
2. Dr. Levin, later Health Scientist Administrator in NIMH and HHS, Mimi Silbert, director of Delancey Street Foundation in San Francisco, and Caroline Sparks, professor at George Washington University in DC, were among those who attended and became friends.
3. With two cans of tuna, two of mushroom soup, frozen peas and macaroni, it proved a winner with three teenage cooks–a five-minute prep, all-in-one meal that began to appear three consecutive nights a week! It had to go!
4. Space doesn't permit a detailed explanation of this technology, which differs substantially from what's now called "interactive TV." For more information, Google QUBE on the Internet.
5. Later the Chief of the Prevention Research Branch at NIMH, and the recipient of the Society for Community Research and Action's Special Contribution Award. Now Joyce Barham.
6. Warner eliminated their QUBE experiment in 1984. Ironically, if the grant had been approved I couldn't have implemented it since QUBE would have been gone.
7. The Stone Center has since become a part of Wellesley's Centers for Women.
8. I am indebted to my friend, Janet Surrey, Founding Scholar, Jean Baker Miller Training Institute, for the many kindnesses she and her husband, Stephen Bergman, Stone Center Associate, showed me throughout my recovery in Wellesley.

REFERENCES

Didion, J. (2005). *The year of magical thinking.* New York: Knopf.

Jason, L.A. (1993). Chronic Fatigue Syndrome: New hope from psychoneuroimmunology and community psychology. *The Journal of Primary Prevention, 14,* 51-71.

Kelly, J.G., Ryan, A.M., Altman, E., & Stelzner, S.P. (1999). Understanding and changing social systems: An ecological view. In J. Rappaport & E. Seidman (Eds.), *Handbook of community psychology* (133-159). New York: Plenum.

Rappaport, J., Swift, C., & Hess, R. (Eds.) (1984). *Studies in empowerment: Steps toward understanding and action.* New York: The Haworth Press.

Swift, C.F. (1979). The prevention of sexual child abuse: Focus on the perpetrator. *Journal of Clinical Child Psychology, 8,* 133-136.

Swift, C.F. (1983). Applications of interactive television to prevention programming. *Prevention in Human Services, 2,* 125-139.

Swift, C.F. (1986). Women and violence: Breaking the connection. *Working paper No. 27,* The Stone Center, Wellesley Centers for Women, Wellesley College.

Swift, C.F. (1992). Empowerment: The greening of prevention. In M. Kessler, S.G. Goldston, & J.M. Joffe (Eds.), *The present and future of prevention: In honor of George W. Albee* (99-111). Newbury Park, CA: Sage.

Swift, C.F. (Ed.) (1995). *Sexual assault and abuse: Sociocultural context of prevention.* New York: The Haworth Press.

Swift, C.F., Bond, M.A., & Serrano-García, I. (1999). Women's empowerment: A review of community psychology's first twenty-five years. In J. Rappaport & E. Seidman (Eds.), *Handbook of community psychology* (857-895). New York: Plenum.

Swift, C., & Levin, G. (1987). Empowerment: An emerging mental health technology. *Journal of Primary Prevention, 8,* 71-04.

Swift, C., & Ryan-Finn, K. (1995). Perpetrator prevention: Stopping the development of sexually abusive behavior. In C.F. Swift (Ed.), *Sexual assault and abuse: Sociocultural context of prevention* (13-44). New York: The Haworth Press.

doi:10.1300/J005v35n01_06

COMMENTARY

Response to Autobiographical Essays by Community Psychologists

Jeremy D. Popkin
University of Kentucky

SUMMARY. Autobiographical essays by five community psychologists suggest that members of this profession often grew up with a strong sense of community and an interest in human interactions, rather than more abstract intellectual ideas. Their life stories reflect the idealism of the 1960s and 1970s that motivated the development of the field. Although these authors have sometimes struggled in the more conservative atmosphere of the past three decades, they retain a characteristic American sense of optimism about the meaning of their lives. doi:10.1300/J005v35n01_07

KEYWORDS. Autobiography, community psychology, family of origin and career choice, social movements and careers in community psychology, private lives and careers

Jeremy D. Popkin is T. Marshall Hahn, Jr. Professor of History, University of Kentucky, Lexington, KY 40506-0027.

[Haworth co-indexing entry note]: "Response to Autobiographical Essays by Community Psychologists." Popkin, Jeremy D. Co-published simultaneously in *Journal of Prevention & Intervention in the Community* (The Haworth Press) Vol. 35, No. 1, 2008, pp. 97-100; and: *Community Psychology in Practice: An Oral History Through the Stories of Five Community Psychologists* (ed: James G. Kelly, and Anna V. Song) The Haworth Press, 2008, pp. 97-100. Single or multiple copies of this article are available for a fee from The Haworth Document Delivery Service [1-800-HAWORTH, 9:00 a.m. - 5:00 p.m. (EST). E-mail address: docdelivery@haworthpress.com].

Available online at http://jpic.haworthpress.com

doi:10.1300/J005v35n01_07

INTRODUCTION

Autobiography is often thought of as a vehicle for individual self-assertion, but the authors of the five first-person essays brought together here use it more as an opportunity to express their commitment to a profession that has given meaning to their lives. Each of these authors tells us some things that distinguish them from others: Irma Serrano-García's identification with her native Puerto Rico, Anne Mulvey's Irish Catholic background, John Morgan's youthful enthusiasm for John F. Kennedy, the family tragedies that so deeply affected Carolyn Swift. But what stays in one's mind, especially when these pieces are read together, are the things these authors have in common, and the collective portrait their essays give of the people who have devoted themselves to the field of community psychology.

Community psychology is an academic discipline, taught by university professors, but, as these essays make clear, it is not for those who wish to cloister themselves in an ivory tower. All of these authors have been committed to activism in the real world. Whereas the autobiographical accounts of members of my own academic discipline–history–tend to emphasize their authors' childhood love of reading and their professional experience of long hours of solitary research and writing, these five authors emphasize youthful patterns of engagement with those around them and careers marked by involvement with communities. "As a child I always saw myself in a helping role," Carolyn Swift writes, and Tom Wolff, looking back, remarks that "as a middle child, I learned skills later useful in community mediation." Education opened up possibilities for many of these authors, but the ethos of research-oriented university psychology departments did not attract them. At the same time, however, these future community psychologists were also dissatisfied with the possibilities of traditional clinical practice. As John Morgan puts it, they wanted to "impact not just individuals but the community as a whole."

Five personal essays are hardly a scientific sample, but these contributions do suggest that certain common experiences helped attract these authors to community psychology. Most came from relatively poor families, and many grew up in tight-knit ethnic communities–"insular, almost tribal," John Morgan writes of his–where solidarity with the group was emphasized over individual striving for success. Morgan and Mulvey stress the role of Catholic social teachings about concern for others in their upbringing. All of these authors report having been strongly affected by the protest movements and the campus unrest of the 1960s. Through these experiences, they became sensitized to social injustice and learned to see collective action as the best way to work for social change. They were, however, quite different from future historians of the same generation, who tended to come from more middle-class families and to attend more prestigious colleges. For historians, working for change was more likely to mean finding a way to remain in academia, rather than an escape from it.

The community-psychology movement, just beginning to establish itself as a distinctive subcategory of psychology in the early 1970s, gave these authors an opportunity to express these values in their work. New and relatively unstructured, the field provided opportunities for young people who wanted to do something different and, as several of these narratives show, it offered possibilities that they might not have had in more established career areas. In addition to personal possibilities, these authors were clearly attracted to a field that emphasized "community," even though the communities they see themselves as helping to create through their work are characterized by diversity rather than by the ethnic homogeneity most of these authors recall from their childhoods.

As we all know, the general climate in American society in the past quarter-century has not always been kind to the idealistic and communitarian impulses of the 1960s and early 1970s. How many other young people engaged themselves on behalf of community psychology in that period but eventually found themselves doing something else is impossible to guess from these essays, which represent the experiences of survivors who managed to remain in the profession despite a hostile environment. In reading these essays, one sometimes has the feeling of having entered a time warp, in which the values and the rhetoric of a bygone era remain alive. Nearly three decades of defensive struggle, dating back at least to the election of Ronald Reagan in 1980, have not made any of these authors reconsider his or her fundamental convictions and commitment to community psychology. As Irma Serrano-García proudly writes, "I learned long ago to follow my convictions instead of my convenience." One is left wondering, however, whether a younger generation of community psychologists who did not share the powerful life-shaping experiences of the 1960s or the excitement of helping to build a new professional field will have the same tenacious commitment to this kind of activism.

Finally, where do these essays fit in the literature of autobiography? Their authors clearly have modest literary aspirations. Although all have certainly written their quota of reports and research articles, they seem less invested in the act of writing than historians, for whom the published book still represents the most important form of communication. Although all of these authors allude to aspects of their private lives that have clearly been of great emotional significance for them, such as the deaths of two of Carolyn Swift's siblings and her decision to live apart from her husband for many years in order to pursue her professional goals, and Anne Mulvey's strong religious impulses and her later acknowledgment of her lesbianism, none of them explores such matters in great depth. The authors clearly understood that these essays, limited in length and intended for a publication that is more about community psychology than about the authors' individual lives, were not occasions for profound soul-baring.

Although the authors present themselves and their field as dissidents from some aspects of American culture, and indeed Irma Serrano-García dreams of seeing her native Puerto Rico separate itself from the United States, their autobiographical essays, like most American autobiographical writing, ultimately affirm many aspects of that culture. These life narratives emphasize many of the failings of American life: racial prejudice, economic inequality, a university system that can favor esoteric research over efforts to improve people's lives. As these authors have experienced it, however, that same society is flexible enough to accommodate efforts at reform, and sometimes even to fund them at public expense. Whatever its shortcomings, the United States remains, in these writers' experience, a land of opportunity for those who have the can-do spirit to pursue their dreams. Between the two great models of American autobiography, Benjamin Franklin's democratic optimism about the possibilities of both the individual and society and Henry Adams's aristocratic pessimism on both scores, the five authors represented here have made a clear choice.

doi:10.1300/J005v35n01_07

Community Psychologists Who Go Beyond the Profession: A Commentary

Roderick J. Watts

Georgia State University

SUMMARY. A "calling" is typically a compelling sense of purpose that arises from a place different from the calculus that leads to a choice of profession. Yet in the case of community psychology, the five people profiled in this essay have both an impressive professional portfolio and a sense of social mission. This essay explores the two sides of their work, and more broadly the challenges facing those who work as agents of change, while at the same time advancing and achieving notable accomplishments in systems that are at once sources of social problems and resources for solving them. doi:10.1300/J005v35n01_08 *[Article copies available for a fee from The Haworth Document Delivery Service: 1-800-HAWORTH. E-mail address: <docdelivery@haworthpress.com> Website: <http://www.HaworthPress.com> © 2008 by The Haworth Press. All rights reserved.]*

KEYWORDS. Profession, social justice, privilege

Roderick J. Watts is Associate Professor of Psychology, Georgia State University, P.O. Box 5010, Atlanta, GA 30302.

[Haworth co-indexing entry note]: "Community Psychologists Who Go Beyond the Profession: A Commentary." Watts, Roderick J. Co-published simultaneously in *Journal of Prevention & Intervention in the Community* (The Haworth Press) Vol. 35, No. 1, 2008, pp. 101-105; and: *Community Psychology in Practice: An Oral History Through the Stories of Five Community Psychologists* (ed: James G. Kelly, and Anna V. Song) The Haworth Press, 2008, pp. 101-105. Single or multiple copies of this article are available for a fee from The Haworth Document Delivery Service [1-800-HAWORTH, 9:00 a.m. - 5:00 p.m. (EST). E-mail address: docdelivery@haworthpress.com].

Available online at http://jpic.haworthpress.com

doi:10.1300/J005v35n01_08

INTRODUCTION

To what extent is community psychology a profession and to what extent is it a *calling*? The two themes coexist, despite the contradictions of working for a cause while having the life and status that *comma Ph.D.* behind your name can offer. It can make community psychology a gratifying–yet peculiar–profession. This outstanding group of psychologists reveal how themes from both these stations in life shaped their values and their careers in what was then a new field of psychology.

Much of the social status of the authors was acquired, in that none of them grew up wealthy. Some families were working class: Tom Wolff, "My father arrived with almost nothing in his pockets." In Anne Mulvey's case, "We lived in a working class neighborhood with little talk of class or status" and thirdly John Morgan reveals "[I was] the oldest of four brothers in a working class family." The families of women had at least one parent with post-secondary education: Carolyn Swift's father "... was a civil engineer. He worked his entire civilian life for the state of Kansas" and Irma Serrano-García's parents in Puerto Rico "... were still struggling to make it on Assistant Professor salaries." Despite these differences, everyone seemed to grow up believing, as Serrano-García said, "It was clear to me then, as it is now, that education was a means to change."

So how are the trajectories of professional and social change agent reconciled? "Careers" or even "public service" would not be the terms we would use to describe the work of those who are extraordinary change agents (e.g., Cesar Chavez, Aung San Suu Kyi,[1] or A. Philip Randolph). Community psychology has not created such people, although at least one psychologist (and priest) Ignacio Martín-Baró has been killed for doing liberation work. On the other hand, all of the writers described how their social values guided their choices of professional activity and the interplay of their work and family life. They are, to a person, activists and professionals, ordering and combining these priorities differently in their very different lives. They used their professional positions pragmatically and effectively to make a significant impact in their fields of interest. Carolyn Swift illustrates her skill in making systems respond: "One of the most serious problems I found at city hall was the adolescent males, most of them African American, who'd been arrested for misdemeanors and jailed alongside adult males–including felons. Some of these teenage boys were being sexually assaulted behind bars. Working together with the leadership of the mayor, the Municipal Court, and the local chapter of the NAACP, I put together state and federal grants to create a residential diversion center for young offenders. Instead of doing jail time they lived at the center and worked, attended school or found jobs."

Everyone drew on their experiences and on their sense of injustice, whether it was personal or vicarious. For both Swift and Mulvey, the insights could be brutally personal as well as philosophical. As Swift recalls, "when I shared with my father the goal of being a doctor, he told me I could never do it because I was a woman." Mulvey said, "I was shocked to learn that my mother had had another last name; I didn't understand how anyone could change something so central to identity. Knowing that women did, but men did not, led to questions about fairness." The experience of domination and the experience of "difference" were vivid in Irma Serrano-García's narrative from the very first paragraph: "I am Puerto Rican. I was born in 1948, in San Juan, the capital city. At the time, Puerto Rico had been under United States (U.S.) domination for 50 years." Although oppression made its mark quickly on the women, they were not deterred. Their fortitude recalls the recent change in the language of trauma: we now talk of survivors and not victims. The marks drew pain but not acquiescence.

The men, both of whom are of European descent, illustrate how social ideals and awareness can develop from vicarious as well as personal experience. In Tom Wolff's narrative, titled in part "My Life as a Community Activist," social experiences in graduate school shaped a commitment to activism: "While in Rochester, I began to explore the social justice aspects of community activism. I did some work in the African American community." For John Morgan, it was privilege (my word, not his) that triggered insights about social injustice: ". . . two circumstances broadened this narrow perspective [resulting from his "homogeneously Catholic" neighborhood]. One I will call political consciousness. I grew up constantly exposed to local ward-level politics, and many of our relatives, beneficiaries of Democratic party patronage, worked for the city." Although words such as oppression and injustice were found frequently in the narratives, it was more difficult to find passages illustrating an awareness of social *privilege*. That particular word never appeared as part of a social analysis, nor did the word "advantage," although disadvantage was used a number of times. "Power" was spoken of frequently in a range of contexts, especially in Serrano-García's description of the Puerto Rican context where domination was palpable. It is difficult for degreed professionals of any race or gender to deny the social insulation and benefits-of-the-doubt that social class–at least *some*times–provides. Mulvey and others mentioned the civil rights movement as an important experience in their development: "TV played a role in my experience of the violence of race. Watching coverage of non-violent civil rights protests was riveting." But it is not clear this experience provoked insights about the *agents* of racial supremacy as well as its *targets* (the same applied for insights on patriarchy and also for heterosexism among those whose orientation was undeclared). The good news? Oppression has entered the field's lexicon. The sobering news? Critical consciousness has its blind spots for all of us, although lived experience sometimes shrinks them; thinking on "liberation" remains off-shore for now in Puerto Rico; dedicated activism sometimes requires sacrifice, something mentioned just twice in the narratives–in neither case was it mentioned in connection with professional work.

Two final points are worth making in an effort to draw some lessons about the institutional settings where careers in the field develop. The ability to create settings is essential for community psychologists who work for social justice. All the people in this group were creative, impassioned, and highly effective in creating places for themselves. It was not easy; a lack of established settings for community psychology sometimes required compromises and professional roles that were more conventional than envisioned. It is a reality of the *profession* of psychology. Said Swift, "What I had to offer were my skills as a community and clinical psychologist. The best strategy, I decided, was to find a position at a Columbus mental health center and integrate [my interests] into a broader set of the center's community prevention programs." Wolff took a "small wins" approach. "I saw that I could make a contribution by encouraging the use of social milieu therapy (on the inpatient units) and of group psychotherapy. Getting a conservative Psychiatry Department to accept group psychotherapy was a terrific learning experience for me." Creativity and compromise were also under pressure from economic concerns. John Morgan confessed to "... soaring ideals about righting social injustice ... and possessing not a clue about how all that could translate into a real job." He described himself as an "applied community psychologist" and not as an activist, and resolving the two paradigms took some doing. "The only unease was a vague sense that, although being a clinical psychologist would be a good way to help kids, this would address only one child at a time and not broader conditions and influences. Ultimately I reconciled this tension ..." Indeed, creativity and commitment had its victories, as García mentions: "One of the first challenges I faced in the program was the lack of practicum settings in communities. In order to place students in community work, I developed a project named Buen Consejo which applied various models ... in particular creation of settings ... The project achieved some change in the community and generated some highly skilled social-community psychologists which continue to be active in the field." Finally, after the creativity overcomes the contradictions and it seems that social ideals will triumph, there are the demands of the family provider role: "Finally, having a clinical practice was a good insurance policy for supporting my family between community jobs."

What are emerging community (and clinical community) psychologists to make of their future based on these narratives? You may not win the next Peace Prize but there is fulfillment and challenge to be had in doing good for society while doing well personally. There are community psychologists who work creatively and pragmatically, yet always with an emphasis on social justice ideals. As this set of narratives shows, even those who do not see themselves as social justice activists can operate within a justice framework as an applied psychologist. Because a doctorate tends to create social privilege and a higher-than-average income, the community psychologist can also live a comfortable lifestyle–or more. Yet there are hazards to reaching for the best of both worlds, for those choosing to see these hazards for what they are. Blindness to privilege, compromises out of self-interest that lead to greater privilege in return for collusion with injustice is a frequent option offered by those in power. This aspect of professional life was not part of the story line in these narratives, but history bears witness to this alternate path. To return to the initial metaphor, settings matter: wells drilled in bad soil can yield tainted water. The remedy: diversity in one's lived experience; unwavering critical consciousness gained though dialogue with trusted friends who share ideals, and for the single-minded, a tolerance for sacrifice. Many examples of this higher path can be found in the narratives of these accomplished community psychologists.

NOTE

1. Aung San Suu Kyi is a nonviolent pro-democracy activist and leader in Burma who, at this writing, remains under house arrest. She won the Nobel Peace Prize in 1991 as well as other international awards of recognition.

doi:10.1300/J005v35n01_08

Reflections on Calling and Careers in Community Psychology

Douglas T. Hall

Boston University School of Management

SUMMARY. The current essay discusses the narratives of five community psychologists from the perspective of a career "calling." Each of the essays highlight different components of a calling: employing deep discernment to know the right path for oneself; experiencing a calling to do one's work, an invitation to which we choose to respond; serving community; discovering your quintessential self or "genius"; and using your gifts for the common good. Moreover, the author discusses how the essays not only illustrate calling, but also the emergence of confidence and the subjective career. doi:10.1300/J005v35n01_09 *[Article copies available for a fee from The Haworth Document Delivery Service: 1-800-HAWORTH. E-mail address: <docdelivery@haworthpress.com> Website: <http://www.HaworthPress.com> © 2008 by The Haworth Press. All rights reserved.]*

KEYWORDS. Calling, career development, subjective career, work/life integration

---

Douglas T. Hall is affiliated with the Boston University School of Management, 595 Commonwealth Avenue, Boston, MA 02215.

The author gratefully acknowledges support for this work from the Morton H. and Charlotte Friedman Professorship in Management, Boston University School of Management, as well as the helpful comments of Marcy Crary.

[Haworth co-indexing entry note]: "Reflections on Calling and Careers in Community Psychology." Hall, Douglas T. Co-published simultaneously in *Journal of Prevention & Intervention in the Community* (The Haworth Press) Vol. 35, No. 1, 2008, pp. 107-112; and: *Community Psychology in Practice: An Oral History Through the Stories of Five Community Psychologists* (ed: James G. Kelly, and Anna V. Song) The Haworth Press, 2008, pp. 107-112. Single or multiple copies of this article are available for a fee from The Haworth Document Delivery Service [1-800-HAWORTH, 9:00 a.m. - 5:00 p.m. (EST). E-mail address: docdelivery@haworthpress.com].

Available online at http://jpic.haworthpress.com

doi:10.1300/J005v35n01_09

INTRODUCTION

What a privilege it has been to listen in on the reflections of these inspired, dedicated, and incredibly caring agents of social change. John Morgan was, in effect, speaking for all of the contributors to this volume when he observed that, "this work has been consonant with my values and ideals . . ." All of this work has been firmly rooted in human values and social justice. For someone who grew up on the writings of Saul Alinksy, Paulo Friere, Carl Rogers, Seymour Sarason, and Abraham Maslow, reading these pages feels like coming home. Yet I am aware of having chosen a quite different path, applying my interests in the field of Organizational Behavior in schools of business and management (with occasional joint appointments in Psychology). So my experience reading these essays has been like a family reunion with cousins after decades of separation.

In addition to the values-driven and social action threads running through these reflections, several other themes jump out of the pages, as well. Perhaps most striking to me is the notion of a *calling* that runs through this work. Even though most did not use this term explicitly, it seems clear to me that their stories illustrate many of the qualities that my colleagues and I have described as part of a calling (Weiss, Skelley, Haughey, & Hall, 2004): employing deep discernment (listening, reflection, prayer) to know the right path for oneself; experiencing a calling to do one's work, an invitation to which we choose to respond; serving community (not just self and family); discovering your daimon (Plato): quintessential self or "genius"; and using your gifts for the common good.

Regarding the first quality, discernment, many of these stories describe in detail the difficult, introspective process of trying to decide what is the right path to follow next or to figure out how to make the right path work along with the realities of life with a partner and/or family. For example, Irma Serrano-García's entire article is a detailed retelling of the various twists and turns in her and her family's journey, as she worked to discern the direction that her *convictions* called for, as opposed to what she called her "convenience." In a similar vein, Carolyn Swift talks about how her long marriage with Bill and their family, with kids in college and respective careers, had all reached a point where it was his turn to "stand by me. I could go [to QUBE TV in Columbus] with his blessing."

On the second point, the experience of a calling–this one is a bit more subtle. Although most did not use this term, several spoke as if their work was a call, which could not be ignored. Tom Wolff talks of being "lured by the vitality of the work . . . " And he ends with a wonderful quote from ancient Jewish writings–Pirkot Avot:

> We can dream of a better world and we can make it happen.
> It is not up to you to finish the work. Yet you are not free to avoid it.

For all of the speakers, though, there is a marvelous theme of serendipity, usually associated with friends and colleagues, in the way they describe the evolution of their work. There is a sense that new opportunities arose out of previous work and associations, and these opportunities were often communicated through deep friendships.[1] Listen to Anne Mulvey describing the way she ended up at the University of Lowell:

> While finishing my dissertation, I took a research job at New York University's Medical Center and did not plan to leave my friends or neighborhood. When Kathy Grady, a friend from graduate school, and Nancy Henley, a friend from the Association for Women in Psychology, both told me that a job at the University of Lowell would be "perfect" for me, I applied despite my reservations about academia. Less than a year after receiving my degree I arrived in Lowell . . .

Or consider the experiences of Irma Serrano-García, taking a seminar with Cary Cherniss:

> This course changed my life because I found a discipline, community psychology, which espoused most of the values in which I believed, but I had not yet seen within psychology.

This process of one piece of work's leading to another comes through especially strongly in the narrative of Carolyn Swift, e.g., work on sexual victimization of youth led to work on blindness to male victimization, which led to the grant from NIMH's Rape Center, which further led to membership on several Rape Center grant review committees and thus to a wide range of new relationships with "many strong women dedicated to preventing sexual victimization . . . " And then, as she noted, "Inevitably our work spilled over into our personal lives and many of us formed lasting attachments." This interweaving of professional and personal lives and relationships is another compelling quality of these stories, showing the wholeness of work and life.

And this gets us to the next element of a calling. These networks of new relationships that grow out of the work create a sense of community around the work. And, of course, by the nature of the setting in which they are doing the work, they are serving the larger community. But for many that is not how they originally defined their work. And for John Morgan, he described this growing awareness of the centrality of serving community as "a progressive change in identity from 'clinical psychologist in the community' to community psychologist."

It is also clear that these stories involve people's choices about how to deploy their skills and other gifts–not just deciding what would be most satisfying or interesting but what would be right, what would be most helpful in the world. As Irma Serrano-García put it in describing how she opted not to pursue AIDS research along the lines being supported by U. S. government funding, "I learned long ago to follow my convictions instead of my convenience."

This process often involved both of the last qualities of a calling: figuring out what is one's unique genius, and what would be the best way to use one's diamon for public service. Tom Wolff talks most explicitly about these spiritual aspects of this work. He leaves us with two questions: "How can our spirituality inform our work for social change? And, how can social change work inform our spirituality?" In his case, he sought the guidance of Rabbi Sheila Weinberg and studied spiritual meditation.

> Through this I began to understand my commitment to social change as part of my spiritual path on the earth. I also recognized that I was not alone in these pursuits.

Not all of the callings represented in these narratives involve an explicitly religious or even consciously spiritual dimension. It may be a more general sense of being drawn to or attracted to a certain type of work, or a feeling that this work represents for him or her what Herb Shepard, one of the "founders" of the field of organizational development (O.D.), called "a path with a heart."

For me these essays show the great value of doing autoethnography, and these essays provide diverse models for all of us readers to see how we can compose our lives.[2] It is also, as John Morgan mentioned, a quite difficult thing to do, as I discovered to my dismay when I tried it, as a way of reflecting on a stint as a dean (Hall, 1995) and then tracking some of my career experiences with the development of the protean career concept that I have written about (Hall, 2003). But here are some simple questions that each of us might consider if we would like to be more mindful in growing in the direction of our own paths with a heart (from Hall, 2003, p. 11). First, have I been undertaking varied projects and assignments over the last few years? Second, do I have a network of relationships that both challenge me and support my growth? Third, have I been consciously seeking learning opportunities? And, finally, have I been getting "up on a balcony" and engaging in personal reflection processes (through a journal, a learning log, a diary)?

A final observation I have on these personal narratives is that they suggest that having a strong sense of mission or calling in one's work seems to convey a kind of support or strength–and sometimes self-confidence–that sustains one through the inevitable difficult periods when one is tested in life and work. Dawn Chandler and I (Hall & Chandler, 2005) have written about a proposed relationship between calling and the emergence of confidence, and these personal cases provide rich data for us to mull over.

In conclusion, then, let me add that personal narratives such as these are just what we need if we are to understand what Everett C. Hughes (1958)[3] called the *subjective career* (the person's own experience and meaning of his or her career). And among scholars of careers, there is a lot of interest in pursuing the subjective career.

> To understand the journey of the self, we must track the more complex world of the subjective career. Moreover, to understand the drivers of a person's career behaviors, we must know more than simply where and when the person has arrived in his or her career. Objective success can be understood by measuring what one has attained, but the deeper sense of fulfillment comes when those attainments measure up favorably with one's own inner purpose. True success is not just getting what you want in life–it's liking what you get. (Hall & Chandler, 2005, p. 173)

We need more self-reflective work like what we have in this volume. And I would call on my fellow careers researchers to savor these wonderful autobiographical essays and to use them to inform their understanding of how careers and lives unfold and grow.

NOTES

1. See Gersick, Bartunek, and Dutton (2006) for a detailed empirical investigation of how relationships in academia can be key in shaping the emergence of careers.

2. More wonderful examples of narratives of academic lives are found in P. Frost and M. S. Taylor (Eds.), *Rhythms of Academic Life*. Thousand Oaks, CA: Sage, 1996.

3. Hughes was the leading scholar of the "Chicago school" of sociology and a pioneer in research on the sociology of careers.

REFERENCES

Gersick, C. J. G., Bartunek, J. M., & Dutton, J. E. (2006). Learning from academia: The importance of relationships in professional life. *Academy of Management Journal*, Vol. 43, No. 6, 1026-1044.

Hall, D. T. (2003). The protean career: A quarter-century journey. *Journal of Vocational Behavior*, Vol. 65, 1-13.

Hall, D. T. (1995). Unplanned executive transitions and the dance of the subidentities. *Human Resource Management*, Vol. 34, No. 1, 71-92.

Hughes, E. C. (1958). *Men and Their Work*. Glencoe, IL: Free Press.

Weiss, J. W., Skelley, M. F., Haughey, J. C., & Hall, D. T. (2004). Calling, new careers, and spirituality: A reflective perspective for organizational leaders and professionals. *Spiritual Intelligence at Work: Meaning, Metaphor, and Morals. Research in Ethical Issues in Organizations*, Vol. 5, 175-201. New York: Elsevier.

doi:10.1300/J005v35n01_09

Index

For Product Safety Concerns and Information please contact our EU representative GPSR@taylorandfrancis.com Taylor & Francis Verlag GmbH, Kaufingerstraße 24, 80331 München, Germany

Printed and bound by CPI Group (UK) Ltd, Croydon, CR0 4YY
08/06/2025
01896999-0002